Transformative Phenomenology

Transformative Phenomenology

Changing Ourselves, Lifeworlds, and Professional Practice

Edited by
David Allan Rehorick and
Valerie Malhotra Bentz

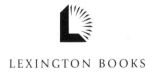

LEXINGTON BOOKS

A division of
ROWMAN & LITTLEFIELD PUBLISHERS, INC.
Lanham • Boulder • New York • Toronto • Plymouth, UK

LEXINGTON BOOKS

A division of Rowman & Littlefield Publishers, Inc.
A wholly owned subsidiary of The Rowman & Littlefield Publishing Group, Inc.
4501 Forbes Boulevard, Suite 200
Lanham, MD 20706

Estover Road
Plymouth PL6 7PY
United Kingdom

British Library Cataloguing in Publication Information Available

Library of Congress Cataloging-in-Publication Data

Transformative phenomenology : changing ourselves, lifeworlds, and professional
practice / edited by David Allan Rehorick and Valerie Malhotra Bentz.
    p. cm.
  Includes index.
  1. Phenomenology. I. Rehorick, David Allan, 1946– II. Bentz, Valerie Malhotra,
1942–
  B829.5.T73 2008
  142'.7—dc22   2008011178

  ISBN-13: 978-0-7391-2411-6 (cloth : alk. paper)
  ISBN-13: 978-0-7391-2412-3 (pbk. : alk. paper)
  ISBN-13: 978-0-7391-6194-3 (eletronic)

Printed in the United States of America

To our students,

who, over the past thirty years,

were tempted by phenomenology

and trusted that we would guide the way

Contents

List of Tables and Figures

Foreword

Phenomenology is many things to many people. In this book, David Allan Rehorick and Valerie Malhotra Bentz show how phenomenology can restore, affect, influence, and change persons, and how transformations that are more than mere influence can happen. The phenomenologists contributing to the edited collection describe themselves and their journeys. They are not mere travelers, but active, participating adults whose transformations can provide insights and attractions that are more enticing than ordinary descriptions. Phenomenology becomes an artful, assimilative experience for those who take it seriously and incorporate its premises, methods, orientations, and perspectives—bodily, affectively, cognitively, and assumptively.

Phenomenology *transforms*, in the word of the co-editors, but more than a word: a demonstration; and more than a demonstration: a presentation; and more than a presentation: a testimony. This book excels in providing detailed accounts by those who have lived and worked with others to bring phenomenology to consciousness; to lived, experiential appreciation; and to incorporation into their own lives. We are invited, here, to read about such transformations as from that of couvade syndrome to cancer survivors, from clinical practice to kidney donation, from empowering Latinas to magically transporting musicians, from studying phenomenology to altering our way of being. In the process of researching others, or uncovering aspects of others' experiences, the contributors were also deeply changed.

In other books on or using phenomenological approaches (such as the various writings of Schutz, Heidegger, Gadamer, and others; or the in-depth studies of particular areas such as disability explored by Goode; or Zaner's examination of medical practice), we are provided with either intense explorations of a theoretical kind, or studies of one field to the exclusion of others. Rehorick and Bentz, however, provide a number of detailed studies, done by different researchers and utilizing a variety of approaches, all of them phenomenological. Their examinations provide us with examples of the ways in which one can go about doing phenomenological research and thereby add to one's own skills in carrying out studies. This book adds in a significant way to our understanding and appreciation of the phenomenological method, approach, and perspective. Various authors do not simply read and then undertake to explicate what and how they have learned. They tell us the process of discovery and research that they themselves have experienced or taught, in order to provide vivid first-person accounts that may also transform us as readers.

One normally reads with a distanced perspective—"So, that's what they were up to! So, that's what happened!"—as though one remains an observer, able to keep distance and thereby avoid entanglements that could lead to discovery of what is lacking in oneself. But this book—by offering numerous studies and detailing the processes of each researcher, as well as providing references and relevant studies that they themselves found stimulating and helpful—engages the reader in a different way. The result is a question that one may pose for oneself: "If they found phenomenology transformative, how am I to do so now? If I have done so, how did I do it? Was it in some of the same ways each writer details, or are there many paths to the same destination?"

This book is of great value in providing assistance to and not talking down to the reader. It engages us in real-life, lived experiences of a great variety, and describes and interprets the transformative process. We can see the "magic moment" in jazz in a way that we have never seen before, or understand how New Mexico Latinas historically have experienced discrimination as they arrive at a new awareness and strive to heal, or find empathic resonance and somatic ways of knowing in new understandings of the self, or find "personal power" as a lived experience in one's being. In short, these authors bring us the vivid, real-life moments to find, for ourselves, that which they are studying.

The transformations produced by phenomenological study and active involvement in reflective phenomenological inquiry are and can be achieved. Rehorick and Bentz, and their co-researchers, uncover and describe these ways, take us as readers on the same journeys, and assist us in finding aspects of ourselves in their accounts. Transformative phenomenology may be the way to show how we can experience renewal—

through our readings, our study, our interviews, our organized protocols, our hermeneutic explorations, our understandings; in short, through all of the mysteries entailed in transformative process—as is shown here most clearly and with great variety.

George Psathas
Department of Sociology
Boston University
March 2008

Preface

The conception and collection title, *Transformative Phenomenology*, springs from our long-term research, writing, and teaching experiences in the domain of interpretive inquiry, with emphasis on phenomenology and hermeneutics. While there are thousands of published books in the phenomenological domain, there is a need to address how phenomenology transforms and enhances personal life and professional effectiveness. This need springs from our observations of what attracts new students to phenomenological inquiry, and sustains their interest over time.

Transformative Phenomenology introduces phenomenological research and practice without requiring readers to delve into the philosophical origins and historical rise of the phenomenological movement. The collection offers an accessible introduction to the field and displays ways in which a scholar-practitioner's life and work may be changed and enhanced by exploring phenomenological pathways and applying phenomenological techniques.

All contributors to this collection have experienced and researched life-world shifts. Phenomenological inquiry enhances understanding of what humans actually experience in their situations and lives. The authors share how their lives, and the lives of those they studied, have been changed through this endeavor. The collection combines contributions from seasoned, university-based scholars with scholar-practitioners who completed their doctoral education in later life, thus blending their workplace experiences with their intellectual interests. This unique mix of contributions expands the scope of interest in phenomenology and hermeneutics beyond the academic realm.

Among the contributors are high-level management, leadership, consulting, organizational development, higher education, counseling, and health-care professionals. All collection contributors display the relevance and power of blending practitioner skills with scholarly intent. Our volume of collected essays can be characterized in these terms: "Phenomenology is our vehicle, mindfulness our fuel, and transformation our destination."

ORGANIZATION OF THE EDITED COLLECTION

Part I, *Coming to Phenomenology: Saying Why and Showing How*, contains three chapters that provide an orientation to the domain of transformative phenomenology. In chapter 1, we as editors, Valerie Malhotra Bentz and David Allan Rehorick, introduce the foundations of phenomenology, phenomenological sociology, and hermeneutics that have had a particular appeal and teaching efficacy among our Ph.D. students over the past two decades. We introduce fundamental strategies such as bracketing, imaginative variations, horizontalization, and effortful possibilizing. Drawing examples from our published studies, complemented by selective illustrations from other works, we emphasize the relevancy of writing rich descriptions of experience as a departure point for phenomenological analysis.

In chapter 2, David Rehorick and Linda Nugent delineate the boundary between phenomenological work and traditional empirical research by exploring *couvade* (a male's experience of his partner's pregnancy). Rehorick and Nugent reveal how phenomenological inquiry about an embodied but unknown experience can elicit wonderment and a curiosity to understand what is happening. They show the relevance of examining findings from empirical studies to offer a more comprehensive picture of the phenomenon.

Sandra K. Simpson, in chapter 3, describes the transformative process that she encountered in becoming a phenomenologist. She explores the fear and wonder of learning to see the world through multiple lenses, and how her life, work, and career were altered in radical and life-affirming ways. Her vivid autobiographical account illustrates the value of a deep reading of historical masters within the phenomenological movement.

Part II, *Lessons from Illness and Personal Trauma: Pathways to Individual Change*, contains three chapters, providing insight into issues of health and wellness. In chapter 4, Dudley O. Tower explores his experience with life-threatening cancer. His phenomenological research, combining his own account with those of other men, led to a shift in consciousness. Surviving a terminal cancer diagnosis led to positive change in his life and departure from his work as a corporate executive. Through phenomenology, Tower clarified the lessons from his experience and embraced wisdom as a way of being.

In chapter 5, Roanne Thomas-MacLean explores women's experiences with breast cancer, using phenomenological and feminist approaches to analyze data collected through in-depth interviews. Women monitored their bodies following diagnoses, and came to view their bodies and culture as traitorous. Her work illustrates how shifting perspectives enhance personal and professional clarity within an ambiguous and fearful context.

Chapter 6 by Jeffrey L. Nonemaker closes part II. His personal story about kidney donation to an academic colleague inside the Greek medical establishment is a phenomenologically inspired account of his personal odyssey. Giving life to a friend became a complex journey, leading to a transformation of how he understood himself and his sense of place as a long-term expatriate living and working in Athens.

Part III, *Empowerment in Workworlds: Self-Other Transformations in Corporate Environments*, contains three chapters, considering how one's ways of working are changed through phenomenological understanding. In chapter 7, Lucy Dinwiddie shows how she uncovered the hidden drama of high-performance teams in international corporations by applying concepts from the work of Alfred Schutz. Dinwiddie's profiles of team members clarify the inner workings of corporate teams. She offers suggestions for more effective and rewarding roles for team participants.

Chapter 8 is Bernie Novokowsky's account of a journey of self-discovery that changed how he works as a corporate consultant. Through the process of writing phenomenological protocols (rich descriptions of experiences) in which he felt the extremes of helplessness and efficacy, he discovers the essence of personal power. Novokowsky cultivates states of awareness that enhance his ability to work with challenging situations in the professional consulting arena.

Adair Linn Nagata, in chapter 9, studies intercultural communication, rising from her experience of organizational change in a Japanese-based global corporation. Her research explores the utility of phenomenological writing to understand, and then practice, *embodied emotional resonance*. Nagata shows how bodymindfulness and attuning to energetic presence provide an opening to the possibilities for change in intense cross-cultural negotiations.

Part IV, *Experiencing Transcendence: Personal Transformation as Collaborative Accomplishment*, closes our collection. Four scholar-practitioners show us how phenomenological explorations of social identity, undergraduate teaching, artistic awareness, and jazz improvisation have changed how they see themselves and their work. In chapter 10, Gloria L. Córdova examines her ancestral heritage and gives voice to Latinas of northern New Mexico. Her hermeneutic expansion of her sense of personal identity empowered her to emerge as a champion of women's rights in her community. She

reveals the paradoxes of pain and joy, anger and love, suffering and transcendence among women of her socioethnic community.

Chapter 11 is a creative breath of fresh air, in which Marc J. LaFountain
examines how his learning of tai chi, along with teaching phenomenology
to university undergraduates, emerged as parallel forms of personal transformation. LaFountain generated themes related to disruption and transcendence, which had relevance for understanding his divorce. In turn, his
explorations enhanced his teaching of concepts and ideas from the work of
Maurice Merleau-Ponty and Alfred Schutz.

David B. Haddad, in chapter 12, describes how he turned his passion for
the phenomenological philosophy of Edmund Husserl into manageable,
bite-size applications that show artists how to enhance their creative
processes. Haddad helps artists to describe and talk about the inner nature
of their work. He developed a phenomenologically based coaching technique, one which transformed his consulting practice.

Our edited collection closes with chapter 13 by Steven C. Jeddeloh. He
explored transcendent states as experienced by jazz musicians in performance, and captures their sense of full expression in the moment, the ultimate high for a jazz musician. Phenomenological inquiry enhances understanding of the experience for the musicians and the audience. He enlivens
the language and methods of his consulting practice as a result of his personal turn into the phenomenological domain.

David Allan Rehorick, Senior Editor
Valerie Malhotra Bentz, Editor

Acknowledgments

We honor our authors for their commitment to phenomenology and their creative projects. We are grateful for their positive responses to our many scholarly prods and editorial calls. Their participants were crucial to the transformational experiences that are captured in this edited collection.

Our inspiration for this volume springs from each editor's scholarly trail, pathways carved from our unique experiences as educators and researchers. David's early phenomenological mentors include Richard Jung, George Psathas, and the late Kurt H. Wolff. Valerie's formative mentors include the late Richard Owsley and the late Helmut Wagner.

Scholars dwell within institutional contexts, and their creative course is supported in many ways. Over a thirty-three-year career at the University of New Brunswick, David had academic license to create and experiment with phenomenological thought in a graduate course. His three-year appointment as university teaching scholar provided essential release time to launch work on this edited collection. Thanks to sociology department faculty and senior university administrators who supported his nomination for this award.

The impetus for the collection arose from the co-presence of Valerie Bentz and David Rehorick as teaching colleagues at Fielding Graduate University. It is no accident that nine of thirteen chapters were written by Ph.D. graduates in the School of Human and Organization Development. They are representative of students who have embraced phenomenology along their paths as scholar-practitioners. We express our heartfelt thanks for the opportunity to develop an educational stream in phenomenology and hermeneutics. We appreciate the personal support of Dean Charles McClintock and Associate Dean Katrina

Rogers, head of the Institute for Social Innovation, for the funding provided to offset copyediting expenses for our book.

Researchers produce; competent copyeditors check and correct. Tangible assistance came early from editorial work by Stephen Figler and Deborah Murray. Preparation of the final manuscript was entrusted to the good eyes and sharp pen of Laura Markos, a wonderful editorial champion. Wan Chang-Hamachi created, painted, and donated the exquisite image for the front cover of our volume. Our publisher, Lexington Books, arrived as a kind of surprise pie-in-the-sky. Gary Backhaus suggested and encouraged our submission, and our first editor, T. J. MacDuff Stewart, responded with enthusiasm and a book contract. Our current editor, Patrick Dillon, and his staff were timely in their responses to our queries, ensuring that we stayed on track. We are thankful for the inspired and mindful attention given to all of the details needed to bring our work into the public domain.

We close our acknowledgements with personal expressions of support.

From Valerie: My work and life are sustained by the pine forest, the ocean, and the wild and tame creatures who inhabit my garden and home. I'm thankful for Peanut, my favorite bluejay, who knocks on my study door each morning, and for the deer who share my flowers. My doggie, Chandler, keeps me down to earth and physically fit due to his demand for walks. My kitties, Lovejones and Spitfire, keep me tuned in to multiple realities only known by meditative cats. My husband, Steve, and my daughter, Pam, provide love, guidance, and support, even when I am preoccupied.

From David: My parents, Michael and Carrie Rehorick, are no longer present to experience the tactile touch of a newly minted book object. Their presence in my life evoked a deep and enduring belief in the value of a good education, and that it could happen to me. Sally Rehorick, my wife, and Nathan, my son, have been encouraging and caring always, supporting my personal quest to seek meaning through scholarship. Sammy and Neville, our current cats, offer fuzz therapy and a presentient consciousness that supports my way of being.

David Allan Rehorick   Valerie Malhotra Bentz
Vancouver, British Columbia   Cambria, California

I

COMING TO PHENOMENOLOGY:
SAYING WHY
AND SHOWING HOW

1

Transformative Phenomenology

A Scholarly Scaffold for Practitioners

Valerie Malhotra Bentz and David Allan Rehorick

Phenomenology, the study of consciousness and its objects (phenomena), is a way of knowing which employs enriched and embodied awareness. Phenomenology directs us to the fullness of experience rather than a remote or pro forma accumulation of information and facts. The creative capacity is enhanced by the opening of vision resulting from immersion in the subject matter rather than limiting the researcher to the traditional mode of observation or data gathering at a discrete distance. The aim of the study of phenomena (objects of consciousness) is to bring about awareness and understanding of direct experience. Unlike traditional methods of research, phenomenology involves the researcher in an enriched awareness of her own consciousness. It challenges one to let phenomena reveal themselves, rather than predetermining what phenomena are. Phenomenology seeks to portray the essential, or necessary structures of phenomena, and to uncover the meaning of *lived experience* within the *everyday lifeworld*.

Phenomenologists use the term *lived experience* to connote the direct feelings, thoughts, and bodily awareness of actual life—what the founder of phenomenology, Edmund Husserl (1913/1931, 1954/1970), called *the things in themselves*. Bentz and Shapiro (1998) offered the following definition of *lifeworld*:

> The lived experiences of human beings and other living creatures as formed into more or less coherent grounds for their existence. This consists of the whole system of interactions with others and objects in an environment that is fused with meaning and language (for human actors) and that sustains the life

3

of all creatures from birth through death. It is the fundamental ground of all experience for human beings. (171)

The adjective *everyday* accents that phenomenology uncovers the extraordinary in the ordinary, and vice versa. Alfred Schutz, a preeminent social phenomenologist, called the everyday lifeworld the *paramount reality*, at once acknowledging that we live in multiple realities and our lives are anchored in the world of everyday life (see Schutz and Luckmann, 1974). Contrary to treating the lifeworld as mundane, Schutz believed that exploring the constitution and organization of the lifeworld provides a fresh and authentic grasp of human understanding.

We have found, through more than sixty cumulative years of teaching and practicing phenomenology, that the deepening of awareness that results from phenomenology is itself a process of transformation. Traditionally, phenomenology had as its goal the elucidation of the true nature of things, in the struggle to recognize the myriad of interferences with understanding. The phenomenological lens is more than a lens of understanding. It is a mirror, which allows the phenomenologist to see oneself in a new way. Phenomenology is a looking glass that is the opposite of the distorted mirrors in amusement park funhouses, although what we see may offer humorous self-insights. Phenomenology clears the focus, reflecting a deeper and truer image of who we are. The phenomenological looking glass also reflects the lifeworld behind the image, revealing structures that we had not seen before, and pathways to new destinations.

This chapter offers a selective intellectual overview of foundational precursors to display our claim that phenomenology can be transformative. We provide an orientation to central strategies and techniques used by all scholars within the phenomenological tradition. We share our own transformative stories to display why we chose to remain within the phenomenological domain. And we discuss how student experiences over time have revealed which entry points and scholars have been most influential in convincing others to embrace the phenomenological and hermeneutic domains of inquiry. The fourteen authors are exemplary scholar-practitioners who have studied change, and changed themselves, through the power of phenomenology. They are all *transformative phenomenologists*.

Our interpretation and applications of phenomenology have developed over time, partly through the distinctly applied context from which many of our doctoral students have come. David Rehorick has worked with the Fielding Graduate University (Fielding), School of Human and Organization Development (HOD), for twelve years, and Valerie Bentz for over seventeen years.[1]

The students at Fielding are primarily seasoned practitioners, mostly age forty to sixty and above, with long careers in fields ranging from corporate or nonprofit management to educational administration, healthcare, community and organizational development, executive coaching, and college teaching. The HOD program at Fielding follows a scholar-practitioner model, one that seeks to infuse practice with scholarly knowledge and vice versa. Phenomenology provides a platform for this fusion precisely because it prioritizes direct experience. Many students choose phenomenology as they seek ways to embrace the scholarly side of their lives, thus bringing practice into balance with the rigors and demands of academic research. What emerges is a particular blend of person-knowledge into what we call *transformative phenomenology*.

We turn, now, to an explication of the features of the scholarship that has fostered personal change and opened fresh intellectual pathways.

EXPERIENCING WONDERMENT

> I was asleep, and it woke me up. . . . I was bewildered because I didn't know what was going on, and I thought somebody was shaking my bed. . . . I looked around and there was nobody. I sat up and I said, "Oh my God, it can't be." You never hear of one around here . . . no way it's an earthquake. I turned on the radio quick, and they had felt the tremors, too, and I said, "My God it was." (Rehorick, 1986, 382)

This extract from the accounts of individuals who experienced an earthquake in an unanticipated location formed the basis for a study that explored how individuals make sense of an unknown happening, a phenomenon that is first experienced as it appears. The turn to meaning-making was clearly a subsequent reflective activity, one that displayed the fundamental phenomenological claim that meaning arises only through a deliberate act of reflection (Rehorick, 1986). It is the sense of wonderment, whether precipitated by external forces or by individual intentionality, which opens a window to phenomenological exploration.[2] Wonderment challenges us to see, to notice, and to take stock of the features of our habituated everyday lifeworlds. While powerful experiences of a fractured lifeworld, like the experiences of earthquake reported by Rehorick, provide one kind of opening to phenomenological inquiry, the practice of phenomenology can be harnessed to render common experiences as special, extraordinary, and worthy of exploration. Max van Manen expressed it succinctly:

> Common experiences require phenomenological attentiveness precisely because they are so common and unremarkable. Phenomenology aims to produce texts that awaken a sense of wonder about the order of what is ordinary. Wonder means seeing the extraordinary in the ordinary. It can only be offered as an invitation to the person who is open to it. (van Manen, 2002, 49)

Wonderment as a deliberate act of curiosity can be cultivated as a phenomenological practice. Phenomenological seeing is appreciative—seeing the wonderment in what is. The imaginative, the hidden, and the possible can also be discovered through the powerful lenses of phenomenology. Phenomenological wonderment helps us to see the spaces in the universe, the freedom of openings, and the opportunities for transforming self, then others.

The accounts and explorations of many of our contributing authors display the power and utility of wonderment. Viewed as a phenomenon, wonderment is an invitation to first ask *what* questions: What's happening? What's going on here? What does the experience look like? What constitutes the essential nature of the phenomenon?

Phenomenology is a return to direct experience as a source of knowledge while rejecting the received knowledge of authority (teachers, preachers, books, parents, history, science, and others). The phenomenologically curious want a fresh start. How does the phenomenologist do this? Simply by starting the journey without evaluating its potential for success (which is itself a form of unnatural binding and self-limitation). The phenomenologist is not, in the traditional sense, a scientist reporting findings. The report is of the journey and its closely observed veracity. The goal is to build up new and fresh knowledge untainted by prior conceptions and evaluations. We become aware of what we have learned to ignore. The end points of phenomenological work are descriptions of essential structures of experience (following Husserl) and/or rich descriptions of lifeworlds (following Schutz).

TRANSFORMATIVE PHENOMENOLOGY: FOUR FOUNDATIONAL PRECURSORS

Transformative phenomenology is inspired by the work of four founders of the phenomenological movement in philosophy and social science: Edmund Husserl (1859–1938), Alfred Schutz (1899–1959), Maurice Merleau-Ponty (1908–1961), and Martin Heidegger (1889–1976). Each of these philosophers has a following of scholars who offer questions and insights into the meaning of phenomenological work (for example, see Barber, 2004; Embree, 1988; Giorgi and Giorgi, 2003; Ihde, 1986, 1990; Moustakas, 1994; Nasu, 2006; Natanson, 1970, 1973; Psathas, 1989; Wagner, 1983a, 1983b; Waksler, 1996; Welton, 1999). We do not intend to demarcate all of the directions and styles of phenomenological inquiry since Husserl. While transformative phenomenology is deeply indebted to this work, it focuses on the ways in which the work of these philosophers and their followers can help the scholar-practitioner bring phenomenology to practice. None of the four foundational precursors practiced transformative phenomenology, although the insights of each of them have indirectly led to profound changes in perspectives of their readers and followers.

Husserl (1913/1931, 1954/1970), considered the father of phenomenology, attempted to ground thinking in full awareness of the interface between consciousness and its objects. Scholars who apply Husserl's phenomenology, such as Moustakas (1994), seek to distill essential structures of phenomena. Uncovering essential structures induces change, but such change is unpredictable (Bentz, 1995b). Since the rise of postmodernism, there is a debate among academics about whether or not essential structures, essences, or *eidos* exist (Bentz and Kenny, 1997). We can set aside, or *bracket*, this question, and still seek to recognize regularities and structures in experience. Experiences and lifeworlds do have forms and meanings that provide the nuts and bolts of our everyday lives (Schutz, 1982).

Taking inspiration from Husserl's later emphasis on the lifeworld, Schutz (1932/1967) selectively applied Husserl's phenomenology to study the social/cultural world. Inspired by Schutz's scholarly turn, Garfinkel (1967) created *ethnomethodology* to explore the underlying processes through which everyday, commonsense activities, and work are accomplished. Ethnomethodological research is inherently linked to practice. However, ethnomethodologists stand apart from their work. They do not address how inquiry transforms the researcher.

A third founding influence on transformative phenomenology was Merleau-Ponty (1945/1962), who established the centrality of the body in experience. Interpretations of meaning are anchored in bodily awareness; histories are sedimented in body cells. Those working in Merleau-Ponty's footsteps engage others and themselves in reflecting on mind-body connection, challenging dualistic concepts such as the classic mind-body split (Sallis, 1981; Varella and Shear, 1999; Zaner, 1981). Yet researchers also tend to offer this work as description and analysis, without reflecting on the effects of the process on themselves or persons or situations under the phenomenological lens (for an exception, see Bentz, 2003).

Martin Heidegger, a student of Husserl, took phenomenology in an ontological and existential direction, focusing on the manifestations of being as it arises and changes in time (Heidegger, 1927/1967, 1962/1977, 1970). He pointed to the nature of humans' existence as the interpreters of being, drawing our attention to the relations between technology and nature. Heidegger's ontology revealed that humans were moving toward a state of existence governed by the forces of a technology that treats all beings as objects of a *standing reserve*. Scholars working in Heidegger's tradition elucidate ways in which our nature is transformed at such a pace that it may become impossible for us to resist (see Ihde, 1990; Zimmerman, 1994).

Heidegger's thinking inspired Hans-Georg Gadamer to develop a method of hermeneutics to uncover the meaning in texts and life. Gadamer (1960/1975, 1976) broadened the field of hermeneutics from the interpretation of meaning in texts to viewing interactions, relationships, and social organizations as texts.[3] Transformative phenomenology links hermeneutics to phenomenology, thus enhancing the search for the meaning of phenomenological descriptions of essential structures of consciousness and the structures of the lifeworld.

Transformative phenomenology, as expressed through the substantive research and personal insights of the authors in our edited collection, draws upon elements of Husserlian eidetic phenomenology; Schutzian lifeworld studies; and Gadamerian self-reflective, hermeneutic analysis. While each of the essays in our collection displays how our authors have applied phenomenology and been transformed by it, we turn, now, to a brief expression of our own origin stories to share our first encounters with the phenomenological domain.

COMING TO PHENOMENOLOGY: TWO ORIGIN TALES

From Valerie Bentz

I entered the path toward becoming a phenomenologist in the 1970s while a Ph.D. student in sociology (Bentz, 2002a). There were no courses offered in phenomenology, but a fellow student and I convinced Professor Peter Munch, a Weber scholar, to offer a readings course for us in the work of Schutz, who brought social phenomenology into the United States and whose work had been translated recently. Like nearly all American social scientists, I had been trained in statistical techniques, including path and regression analysis, mathematical modeling, experimental design, and survey research design. As powerful and important as these methodologies are, I always found myself more interested in what happened in between the arrows in the path-analysis diagrams.

Weber's (1921/1968) *verstehen* sociology (sociology of understanding), along with George Herbert Mead's (1934) symbolic interaction theory, were accepted in American sociology at that time and provided a basis for exploring meaning. What did phenomenology have to add? Schutz thought that Weber had not gone deeply enough into the processes of consciousness as they intend and bestow meaning on objects and events. I found elegance and clarity in Schutz's work: his description of the lifeworld's systems of typifications and characterization of social scientists as making typifications of typifications, creating *homunculae* (puppets). Schutz's social phenomenology expanded Mead's view of consciousness to include multiple realities and levels of awareness—from asleep to wide awake. My first published article used this expanded view to interpret several hundred autobiographies (Malhotra, 1977).

I have researched various topics using interpretive phenomenology over the past thirty years. I have examined the accomplishment of music in a symphony orchestra (Malhotra, 1981), the effects of childhood on women's lives (Bentz, 1989), visual images of women (1993), deep learning in groups (1992), the embodiment of memory and wisdom (2003), and developing a cross-cultural action-research team in Mizoram, India (2005). Phenomenology and hermeneutics became two of the four cornerstones of mindful inquiry, which anchors the social researcher (see Bentz and Shapiro, 1998).

Today, after more than thirty years on the pathway of phenomenology, I know that Professor Richard Owsley, one of my early mentors, was correct when he jokingly warned, "Watch out before you study phenomenology; you will never be the same." My own transformation is manifest by the way that I see each moment as open to various perceptive and interpretive insights. I more routinely examine the preconceptions I bring to a situation, am more aware of the particularity of my point of view, or the way my mood may affect what I perceive. The techniques that we discuss later in this chapter, such as imaginative variations, have strengthened my meditative practice. I've taught bracketing to mentees and massage clients and have seen the benefits (Bentz, 2003). I see phenomenological practice as an antidote to any kind of fundamentalism, whether religious, political, or economic. In a world dominated by wars between fundamentalisms, what could be more needed!

From David Rehorick

I was a graduate student of formal and social demography when I stumbled into the phenomenological domain by chance in 1971. I had been immersed in a world of facts, statistical methods, and census-data sheets when I entered Dr. Richard Jung's sociological theory seminar at the University of Alberta in Canada. There, I was "plunged into a world which intuitively 'made sense' long before I could express what I thought it meant" (Rehorick and Taylor, 1995, 391). I offer selective excerpts from a longer published expression of my entry point.

> "Plunged into" aptly characterizes my first encounter with concepts I could neither spell nor understand—phenomenology, ontology, hermeneutics! . . . Jung's eclectic, interdisciplinary knowledge left me spell-bound as he expanded my intellectual horizons by quantum leaps. This accidental (perhaps karmic) detour thrust me into a world where understanding took precedence over

explanation, and the search for meaning replaced more authoritative asser-
tions about cause-effect-prediction. The more I listened, the more this stuff felt
right. (391)

Without a mentor or suggested way to enter the readings, I set myself a summer project to start reading phenomenological works, beginning with *Ideas
I: General Introduction to Pure Phenomenology* (Husserl, 1913/1931). I virtually copied the dense and condensed thought, since all attempts to sum-
marize fell short of what I sensed to be the fuller meaning of Husserl's work:
"The rational, assured paths of my previous scholarly orientation came into
conflict with the vague, uncertain, and open-ended nature of my struggle
with phenomenologically-oriented thinkers such as Husserl, Heidegger,
Sartre, Merleau-Ponty, and Ricoeur" (Rehorick and Taylor, 1995, 391).

Thus began my career and lifelong interest in studying and seeking to apply phenomenology to the social and human sciences. An account of formative moments in my professional development, ties to the Society for Phenomenology and the Human Sciences (SPHS), and my editorial work with
the journal *Human Studies* are captured in the twenty-fifth anniversary cele-
bration edition of the journal (Rehorick, 2002). The following statement,
taken from my curriculum vitae, expresses the centrality of my first encounters with the phenomenological domain to my research and teaching
over the past thirty-five years:

> My multi-disciplinary research and pedagogical activities are guided by a con-
> tinuing commitment to interpretive and qualitative approaches to the study of
> human experience. One expression is through my philosophical, theoretical
> and applied research, writing, and editorial activity in the domain of "applied
> social phenomenology." The study of human consciousness through phenom-
> enology provides one powerful lens to explore the deep and subtle features of
> human development through expressions of individual and collective experi-
> ence. My work has advanced theoretical understanding of the foundations of
> phenomenological sociology inspired by the work of Alfred Schutz and has ex-
> plored practical topics of relevance in the fields of natural disaster studies,
> nursing and health, and higher education. (Rehorick, 2004)

Intellectually, I prefer to dwell within what I have called *applied social phenomenology*. My orientation is *phenomenological* since I am concerned with
experience, especially that arising from wonderment or astonishment in the
face of the world. My orientation is *social* because I examine the structure of
the everyday lifeworld and the meaning of mundane categories. And my
orientation is *applied* in the philosophical sense of seeking to bring clarity
to a particular event by harnessing the insights won in a more general domain. An *applied social phenomenologist* works with descriptive accounts of
lived experience. Description is a way of accessing modes of experiencing

and the possibilities through which things are given. Much of the ambiguity surrounding the meaning of description in phenomenology arises because what starts as a method becomes a way of seeing (original formulation in Rehorick, 1988). Throughout my career, I have sought to be mindful of Husserl's directive that phenomenology aims to end where the empirical sciences begin. And I have drawn continuing inspiration from Merleau-Ponty's (1945/1962) claim that phenomenology is first about finding its meaning within ourselves (Rehorick, 2002, 471).

Coming to the phenomenological and hermeneutic domains of inquiry has shaped all of my scholarly pursuits and life's tasks. I'm drawn to question questions, and seek to uncover foundational features of everything that I encounter. All of my pedagogical and research interests have been deepened by my quest to see and understand what constitutes their bases. While much of my work does not discuss phenomenology explicitly, there is always a powerful and essential underlying implicit impact. Others who have fully embraced the phenomenological domain can sense it, even if the words saying "I'm doing it" are not always evident. And when my research question calls for a straight-ahead empirical approach, I know that my work is enriched by the tacit awareness that phenomenology brings to all my scholarly endeavors. While critics of phenomenological sociology, interpretive studies, and hermeneutics proclaim that such approaches remain elusive and ephemeral, they fail to recognize and acknowledge that there are well-developed strategies within the phenomenological movement.

BASIC PHENOMENOLOGICAL TECHNIQUES: USEFUL AND PRACTICAL STRATEGIES

Husserlian eidetic phenomenology seeks, through rich description and phenomenological analyses, to *get back to the things themselves*. The *eidos* or essential structure that results from such analysis brings clarity and precision to what an experience is. Some techniques used in eidetic phenomenology are bracketing, imaginative variations, and horizontalization, which we briefly describe here. Beyond their introduction by Husserl, all phenomenologically inspired thinkers and practitioners have applied these strategies widely.

The Utility of Bracketing

The phenomenologist learns to recognize, then set aside, the myriad assumptions, filters, and conceptual frameworks that structure our perceptions and experiences. This process can never be complete as each new situation and horizon embodies change. However, once one has learned to perceive phenomenologically, one can never again take the world of every-day life at face value. While this may initially feel like a loss or problem, the perceptions of flux lead to deeper comprehension and appreciation of one's lifeworld.

Husserl (1954/1970) developed the technique of bracketing to assist phenomenologists to apprehend the essence of an experience and uncover the essential structures of the lifeworld. Drawn from his profession as a mathematician, bracketing means setting aside facets of a situation in or-der to clarify relationships among parts, as in an algebraic equation (256–57). In effect, one puts brackets around one part of the equation (leaving it untouched, only set aside) while working to solve another part of the equation.

George Psathas (1989) offered a succinct commentary on the meaning and utility of bracketing, one that has relevance beyond his application of phenomenology to sociology:

> For the sociologist, a phenomenological approach to observing the social world requires that he break out of the natural attitude and examine the very assumptions that structure the experience of actors in the world of everyday life. A method that provides assistance in this is "bracketing" the assumptions of everyday life. This does not involve denying the existence of the world or even doubting it (it is not the same as Cartesian doubt). Bracketing changes my attitude toward the world, allowing me to see with clearer vision. . . . The so-cial world remains there, ready for examination and description as it is experi-enced. My attitude toward it changes for me, for my purpose at hand is now the examination of my consciousness of it. But I do not deny its existence. (16)

In developing the technique of bracketing, Edmund Husserl differentiated among three levels. Movement through each level leads to increased clarity and fuller understanding. To get at the *whatness* of phenomena, one begins by describing and writing about what one experiences. Bentz articulates the connection between phenomenological descriptions and bracketing:

> Phenomenological description takes place in a partially cleared space. The clearing is created by levels of bracketing. A first level of bracketing is to sus-pend what we have learned about a phenomenon from scientific studies, ac-cepted theories, and other legitimated sources of knowledge. Next one must bracket the notions about the object stemming from one's cultural milieu.
>
> Bracketing is a messy process which is carried out in steps and is always par-tial. The investigator is able to bracket only insofar as he or she can see a sci-entific or cultural assumption that he or she holds in relation to the object and its effects on how the phenomenon is experienced. . . . The difference between a phenomenologically based empirical investigation and a positivistic one is the framework and the assumptions of the two approaches. A phenomenolo-gist approaches an empirical investigation as a bracketing experiment. The

framework is not to discover "facts" but to elucidate aspects of a phenomenon while holding others constant. (Bentz, 1995b, 142–43)

Kurt H. Wolff reminds us that we can only bracket as far as humanly possible, and that bracketing may occur spontaneously or be a deliberate act of our attention. When our traditional, habitual, and customary methodologies fail, we begin to wonder about and bracket them in order to explore our puzzlement and confusion (Wolff, 1978, 501–2). In this sense, phenomenology is a foundation-seeking enterprise, one that seeks to both shore up and challenge the assumptions from which our empirical research begins. Even Husserl recognized that his search for a presuppositionless base for reconstituting knowledge was an ideal rather than existentially real (Husserl, 1913/1931, 1954/1970).

Disabilities are naturally occurring brackets about what is *normal* (Merleau-Ponty, 1945/1962). We can learn much about sight by studying the experiences of the blind, and about hearing from the deaf. Bentz (1995a) experienced something like this with a graduate student, "Paul," who had a writing disability that prevented him from writing in academic style. When he sat down to write, he could only write from a special place and his writing came out in beautiful fiction that illustrated the concepts that a scholarly paper would have attempted to describe. In this graduate seminar, most of the students were skilled writers of academic papers, but they could not master the art of describing their direct experience in phenomenological protocols. Ironically, Bentz feared that she would have to fail the one student who not only grasped but also embodied writing from his direct experience, performing bracketing and imaginative variations in his fictionalized accounts. By dialoguing with Paul about his work, she was able to document that he indeed had mastered the assigned material and succeeded in the course. While Paul could not write academically about the concept of typifications, he could write a story about the important experience of typifications. Paul described his story as follows:

This story is about a boy with a white abusive father who cannot relate. His "uncle" is a black man . . . society cannot allow this relationship but the black man is the "father-in-love" in the sense of father and son . . . the boy has to "bracket" his engrained negative feelings about black people in order to let himself receive this positive relationship. (Bentz, 1995a, 53–54)

Husserl believed that, by setting aside or bracketing aspects of a phenomenon until one could come to its essential form, one would be able to describe it in such a way that others who worked similarly could also discover the same essential structure. There is, yet, a third and deeper level of bracketing wherein one sets aside the object of consciousness itself. Here one experiences *pure consciousness*, which Husserl called the *transcendental level* in which one is aware of the self beneath the particular content of the experience (see Husserl, 1954/1970, 257–65). While this third level has been the subject of extensive debate within and beyond phenomenological philosophy, the utility of practicing bracketing (levels 1 and 2) is widely displayed in research in the social, nursing, and educational domains of inquiry.

Critics of phenomenology also claim that it is a solipsistic enterprise that references only the experience of each singular individual (see Smelser, 1988). However, the applications of phenomenological philosophy to the social, human, and cultural sciences explore both individual and intersubjective patterns. In the phenomenological tradition, the uniqueness of an individual subject's account of any phenomenon is co-presented with intersubjective patterns and themes that emerge from analytical work. The special contribution of phenomenological inquiry is that it honors both unique and intersubjective features as co-present and of equal value (for illustration, see Rehorick, 1986). Following Husserl's directive that phenomenology aims to be a rigorous science, it has always been accepted that intellectual and analytical confirmation by one's colleagues is an essential ingredient of phenomenological inquiry (Natanson, 1967).

Using Imaginative Variations

Clark Moustakas characterizes the process of imaginative variation:

> The task of Imaginative Variation is to seek possible meanings through the utilization of imagination, varying the frames of reference, employing polarities and reversals, and approaching the phenomenon from divergent perspectives, different positions, roles, or functions. The aim is to arrive at structural descriptions of an experience, the underlying and precipitating factors that account for what is being experienced; in other words the "how" that speaks to conditions that illuminate the "what" of experience. (Moustakas, 1994, 97–98)

The purpose of imaginative variation is to shift our attention away from facts and measurable entities toward meanings and essences (98). For example, if I am trying to describe the essence of stage fright in the experience of piano students in recital before a panel of judges, I would consider what the elements of fear in this and other situations might include, such as loss of breath, the feeling of being out of control, and racing heartbeat. Using imaginative variation, I might tell students to envision the panel of judges just wearing their underclothes. What happens to one's description of fear when imagined from such a perspective? To locate the essential structures of fear, one imaginatively changes components with the aim of discovering what must be present and what does not need to be present for the phenomenon to be called fear (Bentz and Shapiro, 1998, 98).

The intent is not to simply imagine and project the bizarre, but to "let our imagination run free, and . . . see what elements we could remove from the thing before it 'shatters' or 'explodes' as the kind of thing that it is" (Sokolowski, 2000, 179). We try to push the boundaries, to expand the envelope of the thing in question. If we can discard some features and still preserve the object, we know that those features do not belong to the *eidos* or essence of the thing. However, if we run into features that we cannot remove without destroying the thing, we realize that these features are eidetically necessary to it. Imaginative variation requires disciplined imagination to go beyond the ordinary and empirical universals that we take for granted, to see what is necessary and essential (179–80).

In his study of an extraordinary experience, which turned out to be an earthquake, Rehorick (1986) used imaginative variations, or what Richard Zaner (1981) called *effortful possibilizing*, to detach himself as analyst from the descriptive reports of his study participants:

> Effortful possibilizing provides a way to detach oneself from the actual by seeking possibilities within the limits of the actual. The identified possibilities may or may not become actualized subsequently. In Zaner's view, there can be no apprehension of what is actual as actual without its being apprehended as one among other possibilities. (Rehorick, 1986, 385)

While study participants used typifications as a way to explain the experience, only a few reports displayed effortful possibilizing in an effort to account for what was actually happening.

> Those accounts that possibilized that it *could have been* an earthquake are especially interesting, since an unknown happening was transformed into a possible phenomenon. Subsequent confirmation by friends, relatives, or the media converted this possibility into an actuality, something which then could be absorbed into one's taken-for-granted stock of knowledge. That the experience was absorbed is supported by the fact that in many of the accounts people did not think about the earthquake after the first day or two. (385)

Building upon insights as to how individuals used effortful possibilizing, Rehorick then explored a range of possible analytical interpretations to account for why individuals knew and then denied that they had experienced an earthquake. His interpretive analysis was inspired by reconsideration of Merleau-Ponty's (1945/1962) assertion that, as long as one attends to the parts of perception rather than perception as a whole, we will continue to make "experience errors" (5). In the earthquake study, such errors are manifest as obstacles to an articulation of exactly what was experienced.

While imaginative variation can be harnessed explicitly as a research strategy, one finds it tacitly used within practices that constitute the organization and structure of the everyday lifeworld. Social phenomenologists are interested in applying this strategy, and in discovering how others may be using it without knowing that they are using it. Those trained in phenomenology are more likely to allow themselves to directly experience events as they occur, an ability that, as in an earthquake, could be a life or death matter.

Practicing Horizontalization

Horizontalization involves making the elements in a situation equal and putting that situation at a distance to better view it without assumptions or bias. Normally, we think of some elements as much more important than others. Horizontalization gives each element equal value, opening up possibilities for seeing things differently and changing one's perspective. Let us say, for example, that in a given hour you tie your shoelaces, pet your dog, write a poem, and watch capsule news on CNN. If someone asked what you had done in that past hour, you might say, "I wrote a poem and watched the news." If your best friend, also a poet, telephoned, you might say, "I wrote a poem." If your spouse called, you might say that you played with the dog.

Applying the technique of horizontalization to these events would present them all as of equal value, maybe even adding some that you had not put on your initial list, such as sitting and staring into space with your thoughts wandering. In this way, you may find that the way you tied your shoelaces was just as important as the memory of the shoes that you used to wear, an idea that became the theme of your poem. The technique of horizontalization could help you recognize that sitting and staring into space is what allowed the connection between tying shoelaces a few moments ago and recollection of your favorite childhood shoes surfacing as an object of consciousness.

Speaking of the process of horizontalization as one dimension of the more encompassing phenomenological reduction, Moustakas (1994) explains that

> Horizons are unlimited. We can never exhaust completely our experience of things no matter how many times we reconsider them or view them. A new horizon arises each time that one recedes. It is a never-ending process and, though we may reach a stopping point and discontinue our perception of something, the possibility for discovery is unlimited. . . . Each horizon as it comes into our conscious experience is the grounding or condition of the phenomenon that gives it a distinctive character. We consider each of the horizons and the textural qualities that enable us to understand an experience. When we horizontalize, each phenomenon has equal value as we seek to disclose its nature and essence. (95)

Valerie Bentz (2005) illustrates the utility of horizontalization in a participatory action research project in Mizoram, India. She worked with a team of twenty North American faculty and doctoral students and more than thirty Mizo partners. They formed a Mizoram Action Research Team that collaborated on projects in the areas of educational change, women's empowerment, and developing a plan to avert *Mautam*, a cyclical famine caused by an increase in the rat population (see Grossman, 2004).

Val Grossman, a member of the original research team, made several trips to Mizoram, at the invitation of the state ministries of education and agriculture, to develop with them an action plan, as the next *Mautam* was predicted to occur prior to 2008. Grossman found that she could not assume that planned meetings would be attended if events which were of greater importance in Mizo culture occurred at the day and time of the meeting. In Mizo culture, church events, sick relatives, broken washing machines, and power outages are routinely given priority over official meetings. In addition, the membership of the committee she had formed in cooperation with Mizo officials kept changing from one meeting to the next. Grossman (2004) found that her training as a phenomenologist was invaluable, as she was able to *horizontalize* these aspects of the situation and *bracket* her expectations. Once she was able to see the broken washing machine as at least equal in importance to attending the meeting, she was able to move with Mizo culture as it was. Consequently, a plan to avert the anticipated famine was developed over a two-year period of time, and is being implemented, rather than having the project fall apart as a result of cross-cultural misapprehensions and miscalculations.

SCHUTZ'S LIFEWORLD PHENOMENOLOGY: TYPIFICATIONS AND RELEVANCE

Alfred Schutz, drawing from the contributions of Edmund Husserl, developed a framework for describing the nature of human lifeworlds (see Wagner, 1970, 1983a, 1983b). Schutz bridged the thought of Max Weber and Husserl in a creative way that brought phenomenology into the social sciences (see Psathas, 2004; Rehorick, 1980; Rehorick and Buxton, 1988; Schutz, 1932/1967).

Fundamental Importance of Typifications

All lifeworlds have the same basic structures. There are stocks of common knowledge consisting of layers of typifications. Typifications are "socially constructed abstractions and simplifications of the complexity of experience that enable us to handle it in a regular, organized, and socially shared way" (Bentz and Shapiro, 1998, 50). We characterize others based on our past typifications of them or persons of whom they remind us. Typifications are mental constructs of attributes about a person or thing, which provide the way we come to know others and objects, based on judgments from prior knowledge (173). The scholar-practitioner who works in a Schutzian mode will make the typifications explicit in the lifeworld and develop typifications of typifications, which Schutz referred to as puppets or ideal-types, to explicate features of the lifeworld relevant to their lives and work.

In David Rehorick's study of first-time experiences of an earthquake as an unknown phenomenon, all study participant accounts displayed the application of typifications from past experiences to try and make sense of what was happening (Rehorick, 1986). Indeed, local newspapers were filled for days with personal reports of citizens, typifying what they thought was going on. The following illustrative excerpt displays how one individual elicited a series of typifications to try to understand what he or she was experiencing. Reference to "the quake" in the opening sentence reflects a recollective account captured on audiotape two days after the earthquake.

> The quake woke me up. At first I looked at the end of my bed and thought it was my dad waking me. It wasn't. Then I thought that it was the washing machine—the spin cycle going crazy and shaking. It wasn't. And . . . we live close to the airport . . . and I thought it was a plane flying low, or heavy trucks rumbling the house. It wasn't any of those things, and then I heard my mom screaming, "earthquake," out in the living room. (384)

While one could imagine a first or original experience as completely atypical, subsequent experiences tend to be compared with and related to remembered features of the first experience. Such features, now familiar, are stored in one's personal stock of knowledge. These stored types shape how one makes sense of unfamiliar situations and future experiences. My personal stock of knowledge at hand is a collection of typifications, sedimented from previous experience and formed according to systems of relevance.

Significance of Systems of Relevance

For Alfred Schutz, the concepts of *typification* and *relevance* go hand in hand (Schutz, 1970a, 1970b; Schutz and Luckmann, 1974). What we see as relevant is shaped by our personal stock of knowledge, an accumulation of our typifications. In turn, our typifications are formed by what is relevant to us, and relevancy is shaped by our tacit awareness of what we think we should be doing with our lives, moment to moment and situation to situation. For illustration, consider the following hallway dialogue that Rehorick, as a university professor, has heard often between undergraduate students:

"I missed class yesterday. Did you do anything relevant?"
"No, nothing relevant. Just a bunch of students talking about stuff."

The exchange ends with an unexplicated presupposition that both parties know what they mean by relevancy, something tied invariably to what students perceive as important for the next class test. In over three decades of university teaching, I have, on occasion, had an absent student ask directly, "I missed class yesterday. Did you do anything relevant?" In such moments, understanding the work of Alfred Schutz has helped me move beyond the feeling of being temporarily dumbfounded by such a remark.

While Schutz explored the structure and meaning of relevancy for shaping our lifeworlds, he noted (but did not develop the ontological implications) that our personal systems of relevance are driven by what he referred to as "the fundamental anxiety" (Natanson, 1971, xliv–xlv). Deep down, I know that one day I must die, and I fear to die. Issues of undergraduate student relevancy about what will or will not be on the next class test are rooted in more profound questions about what I could, should, and need to do with my limited time on this planet. Schutz stressed that the ways in which our everyday lives are structured around various forms of acting, thinking, and being are assumed to be relevant. Mostly, these relevancies are outside our awareness and taken for granted. As they remain unexamined, we act as if they are real or true, when this is frequently not the case. Building upon the work of William James (1891), Schutz clarified that what counts as *real* is whatever one's consciousness attends to at the moment.

The scholar-practitioners in our edited collection encounter a myriad of typifications within their specialized, personal, and professional stocks of knowledge. Whether those with whom you practice are patients, clients, research participants, employees, or criminals tells much about the outcomes of your engagement. If you are a clinical psychologist, diagnostic categories in the *DSM-IV* (American Psychiatric Association, 1994) provide one with typified descriptions, accounts, and outcomes of client and patient action and behaviors. Professionals need such devices to codify their practices. The danger lies in getting locked into believing that these categories are real rather than constructed types. Wiggins and Schwartz (1988) applied and critically extended Schutz's conception of typifications to demystify a variety of psychiatric diagnoses. Phenomenological inquiry displays how typifications can help and hinder professional practice.

Phenomenology provides a philosophical and practical framework for understanding the dialectics between relevancy and typifications and how these and other phenomenologically based concepts can enrich our understanding of the structures and organization of the everyday lifeworld. Phenomenology allows, indeed, requires, one to see clearly where one is going and with whom. It is an antidote to dogmatism, whether dogma by way of religion, politics, discipline, or culture. The phenomenologist learns to reach below the surface. The distortions of everyday life and scientific preunderstandings are brought into the foreground of one's awareness. The phenomenologist as practitioner can then more clearly describe the direct, unclouded experiences about *what is* rather than simply operating with prescribed, artificially constructed categories.

The concept of relevance also plays an important part in understanding how we select and attend to some features of our experience, while relegating other aspects to the background. The work of Schutz (1970a, 1970b) and Luckmann (Schutz and Luckmann, 1974) is key to understanding the relations among systems of relevance, typification, and the lifeworld. While we cannot elaborate these concepts here, we recommend Psathas's (1989, chapter 3) as a helpful introduction.

GADAMER'S HERMENEUTICS: INTERPRETING PHENOMENON

While phenomenology and hermeneutics originated as distinct but co-present intellectual traditions, they are often linked. They are not the same, yet the meaning and application of one are tied to those of the other. Once we have written a description or series of descriptions of a phenomenon, presented the typifications operating in a lifeworld, explored the experience using bracketing and other techniques, we then look at "What does this mean?" As scholars, we will end up with *texts*, which themselves carry multiple possible meanings. Hermeneutics, as the interpretation of meaning in texts, is therefore a natural complement to phenomenology.

Hans-Georg Gadamer's (1960/1975, 1976) vision of hermeneutics is most relevant to the kind of phenomenological work exemplified in this edited collection. Bentz and Shapiro characterized Gadamer's work this way:

> Gadamer sees hermeneutics as a form of play that is an encounter between traditions. Prejudice is rehabilitated in the recognition that we always bring foreknowledge and typifications from the past into the new ones in the present. . . . Gadamer views the hermeneutic space as a place where one reaches out to someone who is a stranger. (Bentz and Shapiro, 1998, 113)

The "stranger" may be one's neighbor, spouse, or even oneself, looked at from a playful yet serious hermeneutic standpoint with the goal of greater understanding. Gadamer (1976) delineated three levels at which one displays hermeneutic understanding. At one level, the interpreter seeks to find universal characteristics, generalities, or abstractions. This level is similar to general qualitative research wherein the researcher finds themes in a text and groups these themes into categories. One interprets an event in relation to the tradition from which it came, such as the practice of constitutional law by way of precedent. Themes can only be visible to the researcher if they reflect aspects of the researcher's culture and history. The researcher looks for patterns in order to see what may be repeated and, perhaps, predictable.

In Gadamer's second level of hermeneutics, one looks upon those speaking in the text as acting, open to being influenced, human persons who may contradict our interpretations of them and make counterclaims (1976, 322–23). In the third level of Gadamer's hermeneutics, the researcher is open to be influenced, is changed by the participant (text), and enters fully into conversation with the other (324–25). A phenomenologist doing third-level hermeneutics reveals his own transformation in the work.[4]

Hermeneutic phenomenology at level 1 is like *seeing* the wild horse. Here one examines the phenomenon and can accurately describe it, bringing the reader into connection with its wildness. In level 2, one is able to *hear* the wild horse as well, to let it speak for itself to the reader. Sound waves penetrate more deeply into one's body than do rays of light. In level 3, one *rides* the wild horse, taking the risk of ending up in a place one did not expect. One lets the horse become the *guide*. It is for us as phenomenologists to observe the wild horses, record their movements, hear them, and even, for a few of us, try to ride them. Few are willing to see wild horses as their teachers. Transformative phenomenologists dare to climb into the saddle.

ENCOUNTERING THE WILD HORSE: FIRST ENCOUNTERS WITH TRANSFORMATIVE PHENOMENOLOGY

Graduate students who encounter phenomenology for the first time often report mixed feelings about the push-pull experience of encountering a new domain of inquiry, an unfamiliar philosophical language, and a methodology which defies efforts to generate a step-by-step, cookbook-like approach. Educators who teach phenomenology and hermeneutics and their applications to substantive areas of research labor to create a supportive atmosphere that maintains balance between the demands for intellectual rigor and authenticity and the needs of neophytes who ask us to make it simple. Hultgren (1992, 1994, 1995) addressed these tensions in her approach to teaching:

> I struggle with my own tensions as I seek to provide an environment where the relatively unfamiliar language of philosophy can be opened to first time students of phenomenology in a way that allows them to not only "know"

phenomenology, but also to experience it as a way of "being in the world" as they "do" the work of phenomenological writing. Comments from students, like the following, bring forward my tensions as teacher in letting learn. "I still want to know what phenomenology is in 20 words or less so I can get on with my research. Even though I know it's not that simple, a nice neat definition would be comforting. No such definition is forthcoming. I guess she's going to make us 'discover' it for ourselves." (Shirley, in Hultgren, 1992, 225)

While many educators resist the pressure to deliver the short-and-sweet definition, some students seek dictionary definitions, sometimes from specialized, domain-specific dictionaries, to satisfy their definitional desires. Rehorick (1995) asked three scholars with long-standing ties to the domains of phenomenology and phenomenological sociology to offer their critical appraisals of terminology related to those domains that appeared in a specialized dictionary, *The Concise Oxford Dictionary of Sociology* (Marshall, 1994). Ronald Silvers contended that the nature of the domain renders questionable the very practice of defining *phenomenology*, and invited us to consider whether phenomenology should be defined or demonstrated (Rehorick, 1995, 417). Elizabeth Behnke responded to the difficulties presented by the dictionary definition's characterizations of *phenomenology* and *consciousness* by reminding us that "what characterizes phenomenology is not a relatively delimited field of objects and topics to be studied, but rather a certain manner of approaching whatever it studies" (Rehorick, 1995, 417–18). Valerie Malhotra Bentz expressed her discontent with positivists who dismiss other ways of knowing, too often based on scanty, secondhand knowledge of the phenomenological tradition. She wondered why the potential contribution of phenomenological sociology to the empirical human sciences continues to be misunderstood (Rehorick, 1995, 418).

So, if it defies simple definition, even challenging whether or not definition is a worthwhile place to begin, what is the enduring appeal of phenomenology and hermeneutics to those who stumble into or are introduced to it in a systematic way? Gail Taylor, a professional writer and poet who returned as a mature student to pursue a master's degree in adult education, expressed it this way:

> Not understanding that what I'd been doing as a writer for most of my life was phenomenological, I experienced a protracted sense of homecoming when I entered David's [Rehorick's] seminar on Interpretive Studies. . . . Although I had not been using the terms of phenomenology and hermeneutics *per se*, the concepts were propinquitous: here was a frame of reference that was capacious, challenging and hospitable to my nature. . . . Phenomenological inquiry, I noted in my journal, was "the art of asking questions . . . encouraging a fabulous curiosity." Responsiveness in the seminar (often in the form of questions) helped to counterpoint what is an occupational hazard for self-conscious lan-

guage-users, who tend habitually to fall in love with nicely articulated ideas in a way that is just as dangerous as what Narcissus did at the reflecting pool. (Rehorick and Taylor, 1995, 392–93)

The contributors to the Rehorick and Bentz edited collection can all attest that, at one time or another, they experienced the forces of push-pull and feelings of hopefulness-dismay while trying to make sense of what phenomenological thinking is all about, how they could apply it to their own lives and projects, and what kept bringing them back to try again and again. Many of the contributors approached the scholarship of phenomenology, hermeneutics, and interpretive studies as a way to begin to make meaningful what they had been experiencing for two or three decades in their practitioner lives We comment, next, on the utility of phenomenology to the practitioner-turned-scholar.

LIFEWORLD TRANSFORMATIONS:
THE CALL FOR A SCHOLAR-PRACTITIONER MODEL

Traditionally, social science researchers have not been concerned with the connections between their work and what happens in their lifeworlds. Management research, like so many areas of knowledge, tends to explore very delimited topics as scholars look for specialized niches within which to make their research mark. There is a split between researchers who are valorized as scientific and practitioners who embody folk wisdom (Gibbons, et al., 1994, 46ff; Buckley and Chapman, 1997). Practitioners often find themselves at loose ends, conjuring up theories and principles on the run. This fragmentation of knowledge signals the need for a qualitative shift in our efforts such that managers and leaders are not just arbiters of technical information, but work from an informed basis, one grounded in human wisdom. Being able to engage the broad range of available knowledge relevant for any practice situation, and make wise decisions about its applicability, is perhaps the most important skill for the emergence of authentic scholar-practitioners.

Bentz and Shapiro (1998) display the centrality of what they have called *mindful inquiry* to help scholar-practitioners "focus on understanding the consciousness of one's self and others and on the accurate and deep interpretation of meanings" (65). They characterized the scholar-practitioner this way:

> To us, a scholarly practitioner is someone who mediates between her professional practice and the universe of scholarly, scientific, and academic knowledge and discourse. She sees her practice as part of a larger enterprise of knowledge generation

and critical reflection. If you are (or if you are intending to become) a knowledge worker or professional, you will most likely be a scholarly practitioner—that is, someone who is continually integrating professional practice and research. (66)

Donald Polkinghorne pointed out the distinction between *techne*, the production of knowledge in order to produce and object, and *phronesis*, the cultivation of judgments to effectively care for the human realm (Polkinghorne, 2004, 114–15). *Phronesis* involves practical perception which

> is a capacity to identify with clarity and discernment the features of a complex situation that are significant for determining the most appropriate action. It brings to the fore aspects of a situation that have gone unnoticed and gives one an intuitive sense of what is important for making a moral choice. (117)

Transformative Phenomenology Is a Way of Cultivating *Phronesis*

As an adult learner with professional practice, personal growth, and intellectual development goals, the ideal scholar-practitioner interrelates concepts, understandings, and methods from varied theoretical and practice perspectives. The fully developed adult professional shows the capacity for emotional intelligence and use of self that reflect tolerance of difference and ambiguity that are linked with compassion for life and a commitment to improving the human condition (McClintock, 2004, 393–96). Most of all, the ideal of the scholar-practitioner embodies and displays wisdom:

> The concept of wisdom captures the essence of the ideal of the scholar practitioner, in that it represents an integration of cognitive, affective, and behavioral dimensions. The work of wisdom for a scholar practitioner requires alternating between the abstract and the observable, questioning what is taken for granted and overlooked, complicating with unexpected findings, and simplifying with new interpretations. These intellectual and social skills require multiple forms of intelligence and are manifested through principled and ethical action. Nurturing the capacity for wisdom is the goal of education and lies at the heart of the scholar practitioner ideal. (396)

Phenomenology provides a philosophical and practical framework for cultivating wisdom by challenging researchers and practitioners to look deeply into their subject matter and themselves. Phenomenology allows, indeed requires, one to see clearly where one is going and with whom. It is an antidote to dogmatism, whether by way of religion, politics, culture, or disciplinary specialization. A phenomenologist must learn to reach below the surface to expose the distortions within everyday life and the trappings of scientific preunderstandings. The phenomenologist seeks to describe experience in direct and unclouded ways.

The practice of transformative phenomenology begins with an exploration of the nature of a phenomenon using an eidetic (Husserlian) approach and a (Schutzian) description of the lifeworld in which the phenomenon appears. Helmut Wagner astutely described these two sides of phenomenological work (Wagner, 1970, 1983a, 1983b). Some phenomenologists emphasize one of these aspects to the exclusion of the other. We contend that, regardless of the ultimate research methodology or practice technology used in a particular study, a preliminary analysis of the essential structure of an experience of consciousness and the structures of the lifeworld(s) in which it occurs is invaluable. In addition, we emphasize inclusion of embodied aspects of consciousness.

Phenomenologically trained scholar-practitioners are well positioned to work in our challenging times. The Husserlian tradition of essential or eidetic phenomenology trains them to find what is central to a situation or experience. The application of Schutzian social phenomenology offers them insights into the structures of manifest lifeworlds. Such scholar-practitioners, for instance, can better understand phenomena such as organizational downsizing by uncovering implicit stocks of knowledge, systems of tacit typifications used to explain change, and the use of effortful possibilizing to see what is lost when organizational lifeworlds are torn asunder. Finally, scholar-practitioners of transformative phenomenology are prepared to ride the wild horse, as they interpret the meaning of the phenomena they study. They experience deep change in themselves as they gain greater agility and skill as riders. Eventually, the wild horse of phenomenology becomes a friend and daily companion on life's journeys.

RIDERS OF THE WILD HORSE: HIGHLIGHTING THE LESSONS FROM OUR AUTHORS

The fourteen authors in this collection share how their lives and work have been powerfully changed through scholarly phenomenological inquiry. They work in diverse professional fields including high-level management, leadership, consulting, organizational development, counseling, healthcare, and postsecondary education. All of the authors found purpose and meaning through mindful inquiry[5] into the events of their lives and topics of investigation. Several helped to bring about transformations in organizations and institutions through striving to reform thought and reassessing or redefining conditions and events. All have brought about transformations to themselves, something that has changed how they see themselves and how they approach the world.

The authors in this edited collection illustrate the ways in which scholar-practitioners can understand, appreciate, and preserve lifeworlds, leading us through stormy times as we search for more effective and wise ways of being, knowing, and working. By sharing their insights and stories, contributors to this collection seek to encourage others to sample the phenomenological domain and come to understand what one can discover and how it can support transformational change to one's way of being in the world.

Taken as a whole, all thirteen chapters offer readers rich, personal, and research-based examples of why a hands-on practice of phenomenology, hermeneutics, and interpretive inquiry is a legitimate and, indeed, necessary mode of inquiry. The essays show the interplay between the worlds of scholar and practitioner, and how movement from practitioner to scholar and back to practitioner augments the quality of understanding and being in the world. The collection supports the claim that phenomenological inquiry is an inherently practical activity, and that the model of the scholar-practitioner is an essential educational mission for the twenty-first century.

While working through final changes to the collection chapters, we as co-editors stumbled across a statement by Edmund Husserl that was remarkably predictive of what we, independently, have come to call *transformative phenomenology*:

> Perhaps it will even become manifest that the total phenomenological attitude and the epoche belonging to it are destined in essence to effect, at first, a complete personal transformation, comparable in the beginning to a religious conversion, which then, however, over and above this, bears within itself the significance of the greatest existential transformation which is assigned as a task to mankind as such. (Husserl, 1954/1970, 137)

The scholarly expression of the professional and personal lifeworlds of our authors testifies to the prescience of Husserl's words. Phenomenology is inherently transformative.

NOTES

1. While the distinct emphasis that we call *transformative phenomenology* arises out of our experiences at Fielding, both of us have had broader and longer term involvement with phenomenological inquiry. Rehorick has offered graduate seminars in the domain over a thirty-year period as professor of sociology at the University of New Brunswick in Canada. Likewise, Bentz taught phenomenology and hermeneutics at Texas Woman's University before joining Fielding.

2. The use of *wonderment* is preferred to *wonder* since wonderment refers to *a cause of or occasion for wonder*. Phenomenology gives rise to an occasion to wonder about whatever phenomenon presents itself.

3. The connection between phenomenology and hermeneutics is a much larger story, one that we cannot develop here. The work of Ricoeur (1981, 1986/1991) is formative (also see Bauman, 1978). At Fielding, we have found that Gadamer's work resonates with dissertation students since they have more readily sensed how they might apply his concepts and methods to deepen their understanding and research abilities.

4. See Turner (2003) for an excellent explication of how to do the three analytical turns outlined in Gadamer's work. Wing (1999) displayed how the three levels work in her study that explored the relationships between doctoral dissertation chairpersons and their mentees.

5. Bentz and Shapiro (1998) and Bentz (2002b) characterize *mindful inquiry* as an approach to research and practice. The mindful scholar-practitioner works with phenomenology, hermeneutics, critical theory, and Buddhist principles of knowing as a way of solidly grounding the work at a time of epistemological disjuncture in the social and human sciences.

REFERENCES

American Psychiatric Association. (1994) *Diagnostic and Statistical Manual of Mental Disorders (DSM-IV*, fourth ed.). Washington, DC: Author.

Barber, Michael D. (2004) *The Participating Citizen: A Biography of Alfred Schutz*. Albany: State University of New York Press.

Bauman, Zygmunt. (1978) *Hermeneutics and Social Science: Approaches to Understanding*. London: Hutchinson.

Barthes, Roland. (1990) *The Fashion System* (M. Ward and R. Howard, trans.). Berkeley: University of California Press.

Bentz, Valerie Malhotra. (1989) *Becoming Mature: Childhood Ghosts and Spirits in Adult Life*. New York: Aldine de Gruyter.

———. (1992) Deep Learning Groups: Combining Emotional and Intellectual Learning. *Clinical Sociological Review, 10*, 71–89.

———. (1993) How Women Look: Critique of Visual Images. In Valerie Malhotra and P. Mayes (eds.), *Visual Images of Women in the Arts and Mass Media* (1–16). New York: Mellon.

———. (1995a) Husserl, Schutz, Paul and Me: Reflections on Writing Phenomenology. *Human Studies, 18*(1), 41–62.

———. (1995b) Experiments in Husserlian Phenomenological Sociology. *Studies in Symbolic Interactionism, 17*, 133–61.

———. (2002a) From Playing Child to Aging Mentor: The Role of *Human Studies* in My Development as a Scholar. *Human Studies, 25*(4), 499–506.

———. (2002b) The Mindful Scholar-Practitioner. *Scholar Practitioner Quarterly, 1*(1), 7–21.

———. (2003) The Body's Memory, the Body's Wisdom. In M. Itkonen and G. Backhaus (eds.), *Lived Images: Mediations in Experience, Life-World and I-hood* (158–86). Jyvaskyla, Finland: University of Jyvaskyla Press.

———. (2005) *Towards "Tlawmngaihna": Participatory Action Research in Mizoram, India*. Unpublished Manuscript.

Bentz, Valerie Malhotra, and Wade Kenny. (1997) "Body-as-World": Kenneth Burke's Answer to the Postmodernist Charges against Sociology. *Sociological Theory, 15*(1), 82–96.

Bentz, Valerie Malhotra, and Jeremy J. Shapiro. (1998) *Mindful Inquiry in Social Research*. Thousand Oaks, CA: Sage.

Buckley, P. J., and M. Chapman. (1997) The Use of Natural Categories in Management Research. *British Journal of Management, 8*(4), 283–99.

Embree, Lester (ed.). (1988) *Worldly Phenomenology: The Continuing Influence of Alfred Schutz on North American Social Science*. Washington, DC: Center for Advanced Research in Phenomenology and University Press of America.

Gadamer, Hans-Georg. (1960/1975) *Truth and Method*. New York: Seabury Press.

———. (1976) *Philosophical Hermeneutics* (D. E. Linge, trans.). Berkeley: University of California Press.

Garfinkel, Harold. (1967) *Studies in Ethnomethodology*. Englewood Cliffs, NJ: Prentice Hall.

Gibbons, Michael, Camille Limoges, Helga Nowotny, and Simon Schwartzman. (1994). *The New Production of Knowledge: The Dynamics of Science and Research in Contemporary Societies*. London: Sage.

Giorgi, Amedeo P., and B. M. Giorgi. (2003) The Descriptive Phenomenological Psychological Method. In P. M. Camic, J. E. Rhodes, and L. Yardley (eds.), *Qualitative Research in Psychology: Expanding Perspectives in Methodology and Design* (243–73). Washington, DC: American Psychological Association.

Grossman, Valerie. (2004) *Preventing Mautam: Phenomenology and Participatory Action Research in Mizoram, India*. Unpublished Ph.D. Dissertation. Santa Barbara, CA: Fielding Graduate University.

Heidegger, Martin. (1927/1967) *Being and Time* (J. Macquarrie and E. Robinson, trans.). Oxford: Basil Blackwell.

———. (1962/1977) *The Question Concerning Technology* (W. Lovitt, trans.). New York: Harper.

———. (1970) The Idea of Phenomenology. *The New Scholasticism, 44*(3), 325–44.

Hultgren, Francine H. (1992) The Transformative Power of "Being With" Students in Teaching. In L. Peterat and E. Vaines (eds.), *Lives and Plans: Signs for Transforming Practice. 12th Annual Yearbook. Teacher Education Section, American Home Economics Association* (221–42). Mission Hills, CA: Glencoe.

———. (1994) Interpretive Inquiry as a Hermeneutics of Practice. *Journal of Vocational Home Economics and Education, 12*(1), 12–25.

———. (1995) The Phenomenology of "Doing" Phenomenology: The Experience of Teaching and Learning Together. *Human Studies, 18*(4), 371–87.

Husserl, Edmund. (1913/1931) *Ideas: General introduction to Pure Phenomenology* (W. R. Boyce Gibson, trans.). London: George Allen & Unwin.

———. (1954/1970) *The Crisis of European Sciences and Transcendental Phenomenology: An Introduction to Phenomenological Philosophy* (David Carr, trans.). Evanston, IL: Northwestern University Press.

Ihde, Don. (1986) *Experimental Phenomenology: An Introduction*. Albany: State University of New York Press.

———. (1990). *Technology and the Lifeworld: From Garden to Earth*. Bloomington: Indiana University Press.

James, William. (1891). *The Principles of Psychology* (vols. I and II). New York: Henry Holt.

Malhotra, Valerie. (1977) Relating to Mead's Model of Self and Phenomenology: An Empirical Analysis. *The Wisconsin Sociologist*, 14(1), 8–24.

———. (1981). The Social Accomplishment of Music in a Symphony Orchestra: A Phenomenological Analysis. *Qualitative Sociology*, 4(2), 102–25.

Marshall, Gordon. (1994) *The Concise Oxford Dictionary of Sociology*. New York: Oxford University Press.

McClintock, Charles. (2004) The Scholar-Practitioner Model. In A. Distefano, K. E. Rudestam, and R. J. Silverman (eds.), *Encyclopedia of Distributed Learning* (393–96). Thousand Oaks, CA: Sage.

Mead, George H. (1934) *Mind, Self and Society*. Chicago: University of Chicago Press.

Merleau-Ponty, Maurice. (1945/1962) *Phenomenology of Perception* (C. Smith, trans.). London: Routledge & Kegan Paul.

Moustakas, Clark. (1994) *Phenomenological Research Methods*. Thousand Oaks, CA: Sage.

Nasu, Hisashi. (2006) *A Continuing Dialogue with Alfred Schutz*. Alfred Schutz Memorial Lecture, Presented at the Annual Meetings of the Society for Phenomenology and the Human Sciences. Philadelphia, October 2006.

Natanson, Maurice. (1967) Phenomenology as a Rigorous Science. *International Philosophical Quarterly*, 7, 5–20.

———. (1970) *The Journeying Self: A Study in Philosophy and Social Role*. Reading, MA: Addison-Wesley.

———. (1971) Introduction. In M. Natanson (ed.), *Alfred Schutz, Collected Papers* (Vol. 1, xxv–xlvii). The Hague, The Netherlands: Martinus Nijhoff.

———. (1973) *Edmund Husserl: Philosopher of Infinite Tasks*. Evanston, IL: Northwestern University Press.

Pert, Candace B. (1997) *Molecules of Emotion*. New York: Scribner.

Polkinghorne, Donald E. (2004) *Practice and the Human Sciences: The Case for a Judgment-Based Practice of Care*. Albany: State University of New York.

———. (2004) Alfred Schutz's Influence on American Sociologists and Sociology. *Human Studies*, 27(1), 1–35.

Psathas, George. (1989) *Phenomenology and Sociology: Theory and Research*. Washington, DC: Center for Advanced Research in Phenomenology and University Press of America.

Rehorick, David. (1980) Schutz and Parsons: Debate or Dialogue? *Human Studies*, 3(4), 347–55.

———. (1981) Subjective Origins, Objective Reality: Knowledge Legitimation and the TM Movement. *Human Studies*, 4(4), 339–57.

———. (1986) Shaking the Foundations of Lifeworld: A Phenomenological Account of an Earthquake Experience. *Human Studies*, 9(4), 379–91.

———. (1988) Accounting for Unusual Experiences: A Study in Applied Phenomenology. Invited public address, Ontario Institute for Studies in Education, University of Toronto, Ontario, Canada, April 3.

———. (1991) Pickling Human Geography: The Souring of Phenomenology in the Human Sciences. *Human Studies, 14*(4), 359–69.

———. (1995) Dictionary Definitions of a Domain: Three Critical Appraisals. In D. Rehorick (ed.), Teaching Phenomenologically: Bringing Others to a New Domain. *Human Studies,* 18(4), 367–414.

———. (2002) I/Human Studies. *Human Studies, 25*(4), 435–39.

———. (2004) Unpublished Curriculum Vitae (C.V.), Department of Sociology, University of New Brunswick, Fredericton, Canada.

Rehorick, David, and William Buxton. (1988) Recasting the Schutz-Parsons Dialogue: The Hidden Participation of Eric Voegelin. In L. Embree (ed.), *Worldly Phenomenology: The Continuing Influence of Alfred Schutz on North American Human Science* (151–69). Washington, DC: The Center for Advanced Research in Phenomenology and University Press of America.

Rehorick, David, and Gail Taylor. (1995) Thoughtful Incoherence: First Encounters with the Phenomenological-Hermeneutical Domain. *Human Studies, 18*(4), 389–414.

Ricoeur, Paul. (1981) *Hermeneutics and Human Sciences: Essays on Language, Action and Interpretation* (J. B. Thompson, ed. and trans.). Cambridge: Cambridge University Press.

———. (1986/1991) *From Text to Action: Essays in Hermeneutics II* (K. Blamey and J. B. Thompson, trans.). Evanston, IL: Northwestern University Press.

Sallis, John (ed.). (1981) *Merleau-Ponty: Perception, Structure, Language.* Atlantic Highlands, NJ: Humanities Press.

Schutz, Alfred. (1932/1967) *The Phenomenology of the Social World* (G. Walsh and F. Lehnert, trans.). Evanston, IL: Northwestern University Press.

———. (1970a) *On Phenomenology and Social Relations* (H. Wagner, ed.). Chicago: University of Chicago Press.

———. (1970b) *Reflections on the Problem of Relevance* (R. M. Zaner, ed.). New Haven, CT: Yale University Press.

———. (1982) *Lifeforms and Meaning Structures* (H. Wagner, trans.). Boston: Routledge.

Schutz, Alfred, and Thomas Luckmann. (1974) *The Structures of the Life-World* (R. M. Zaner and H. T. Englehardt, trans.). London: Heinemann.

Smelser, Neil J. (ed.). (1988) *Handbook of Sociology.* Beverly Hills, CA: Sage.

Sokolowski, Robert. (2000) *Introduction to Phenomenology.* New York: Cambridge University Press.

Turner, de Sales. (2003) Horizons Revealed: From Methodology to Method [Electronic Version]. *International Journal of Qualitative Methods, 2*(1), 1–10.

van Manen, Max. (1997). *Researching Lived Experience: Human Science for an Action Sensitive Pedagogy* (second ed.). London, Ontario, Canada: Althouse Press.

———. (2002) Common Experiences. In Max van Manen (ed.), *Writing in the Dark: Phenomenological Studies in Interpretive Inquiry* (49–60). London, Ontario, Canada: Althouse Press.

Varella, Francisco, and Jonathan Shear (eds.). (1999) *The View from Within: First-person Approaches to the Study of Consciousness.* Bowling Green, OH: Imprint Academic.

Wagner, Helmut. (1970) Introduction. In H. Wagner (ed.), *Alfred Schutz: On Phenomenology and Social Relations* (1–50). Chicago: University of Chicago Press.

———. (1983a) *Alfred Schutz: An Intellectual Biography*. Chicago: University of Chicago Press.

———. (1983b) *Phenomenology of Consciousness and Sociology of the Lifeworld: An Introductory Study*. Edmonton, Alberta, Canada: University of Alberta Press.

Waksler, Frances Chaput. (1996) *The Little Trials of Childhood and Children's Strategies for Dealing with Them*. London: Falmer Press.

Weber, Max. (1921/1968) *Economy and Society* (three vols.). In G. Roth and C. Wittich (eds.). Totowa, N.J.: Bedminister Press.

Welton, Don. (1999) The Development of Husserl's Phenomenology. In Don Welton (ed.), *The Essential Husserl: Basic Writings in Transcendental Phenomenology* (ix–xv). Bloomington: Indiana University Press.

Wiggins, Osborne P., and Michael A. Schwartz. (1988) Psychiatric Diagnosis and the Phenomenology of Typification. In Lester Embree (ed.), *Worldly Phenomenology: The Continuing Influence of Alfred Schutz on North American Human Science* (203–30). Washington, DC: Center for Advanced Research in Phenomenology and University Press of America.

Wing, Linda. (1999) *Transforming Doctoral Candidates: An Exploration of Faculty Student Relations Through Dissertation Creation*. Unpublished Ph.D. Dissertation, Fielding Graduate Institute, Santa Barbara, CA.

Wolff, Kurt H. (1978) *Phenomenology and Sociology*. In T. Bottomore and R. Nisbet (eds.), *A History of Sociological Analysis* (499–556). New York: Basic Books.

Zaner, Richard. (1981) *The Control of Self: A Phenomenological Inquiry Using Medicine as a Clue*. Athens, OH: University of Ohio Press.

Zimmerman, Michael E. (1994) *Contesting Earth's Future: Radical Ecology and Postmodernity*. Berkeley: University of California Press.

2

Male Experiences of Pregnancy

Bridging Phenomenological and Empirical Insights

David Allan Rehorick and Linda Nugent

> During a business trip, I experienced swelling in both feet, followed by stiffness in my hands and fingers. Within a week, the problem had intensified and I could not strap on sandals. I thought that my swelling was caused by hot and humid weather. I also wondered if the toxic chemicals that I had recently been using might have had some effect. When I returned home, I learned that Sally had experienced fluid build-up in her feet and ankles. I was surprised by the fact that the problem extended to her hands and fingers. (David Rehorick, personal diary/fieldnotes)

This descriptive excerpt is drawn from a more comprehensive personal account of David Rehorick's first-time experience with the pregnancy and childbirth process. For several months during 1983, David experienced a wide array of bodily sensations and physical symptoms that he eventually realized were somehow connected to his wife Sally's experience during pregnancy, labor, and childbirth. David had neither name nor knowledge to explain what was going on, but trusted his phenomenological training and scholarship to help him track the embodied trail which was unfolding in a vague yet evident way. Phenomenology teaches us that what's first felt is only later understood, and that what's experienced calls for a descriptive effort to begin the meaning-making process.

This chapter displays the practical utility of using a phenomenological orientation to track and explore one's lived experience. Phenomenology offers a preconceptual way to grasp the lived experience of a phenomenon that one cannot yet label or name. As such, phenomenology provides access to the wonderment of world and being before any attempt is made to examine that world from an empirical and scientific stance. Drawing selectively from the descriptive accounts kept by David during the pregnancy phase of Sally's childbirth process, this chapter reveals how an originally unknown experience begins to take shape and form in a manner that remains close to the lived experience itself. Then, the discussion turns to what was discovered through a review of the empirical research literature of what's been called *couvade*. The intent is to display that, contrary to the claims by many readers and researchers, phenomenology and empirical studies are not oppositional. When combined, the insights of phenomenological inquiry and the results of empirical studies offer a fuller and richer understanding of the phenomenon under consideration. The chapter closes with a commentary by Linda Nugent as to how and why her turn to phenomenology and interpretive studies transformed how she thinks and conducts research.

EMBODIED WONDERMENT:
EXPERIENCING THE UNNAMED LIFEWORLD

Wonderment is a phenomenological opening to experiencing the fullness of life and world, even when one cannot name, or label, or place what's happening. In a systematic series of personal diary (field)notes, written over the course of my wife's pregnancy, labor, and childbirth, I traced how unusual alterations to habituated bodily patterns made me aware of possible connections to Sally's pregnancy pains. Since I had no knowledge of research related to this phenomenon of couvade, my understanding sprang from a watchful curiosity about what was happening.

I tape-recorded the full descriptive account, both retrospective and prospective, between June 20 and July 27, 1983, with the birth of our son, Nathan Paul, occurring on July 24. I also kept written notes on a variety of experiences during the course of Sally's pregnancy. One year later (July 1984), I transcribed the account (seventy double-spaced pages), organized it thematically, and edited it for clarity. I indexed the transcriptions using the following thematic scheme:

- *Sympathetic symptoms (physical)*, including back pains, swelling, headache, leg cramps, stomach cramps, and breast firmness;
- *Sympathetic symptoms (psychological)*, including depression, mood swings, imagined sense of being pregnant, and breast-feeding;
- *Expressed fears*, including delivery room, trust in medical staff, quality of support to partner, lack of preparation for features of experience, loss of personal solitude, and holding the baby; and
- *Reactions to/reflections on birth*, including first contact with baby, size of head, placenta and cord, establishing baby's identity, repression of

pain/release of emotion, perception of wife's experience of pain/joy, my perception of contractions as negative, and perceptions of spouse before and after the birth.

Once the indexing task was completed, I generated summary statements that pulled thematic material together. Lastly, I crosschecked my notes with Sally's personal diary. I did not access or request to see her account until several months after the birth. Sally's written record ended in March of 1983, toward the end of the second trimester. A fall, resulting in a deep cut in her right hand, meant that she was unable to write for several months. I had become aware of the possibility of some kind of connection, but had no way of accounting for what I felt. Below, I offer three excerpts from my descriptive accounts to display how a sense of embodied connection unfolded.

Data Excerpt #1

Although I suspected a link between the backaches, which Sally and I experienced during the first trimester of her pregnancy, I also doubted the connection. A first indication of possible bodily response to my wife's physical symptoms was our communication and thus discovery that we had both been experiencing similar back pains:

> The exact starting date cannot be specified. What is interesting is that we feel that we began about the same time, but did not want to complain of problems to each other. I noted later in my field notes that I have had back pains in the past; therefore, it would be difficult to specify whether or not they were related to pregnancy or other factors.

I accounted for symptoms such as backache, headache, and stomachache as either responses to stress or consequences of altered sleeping patterns. It was only during the last five weeks of the pregnancy, when the intensity and range of symptoms increased, that I began to record, in much more detail, what was occurring.

Data Excerpt #2

One reason that men fail to recognize the connection is that symptoms such as gastrointestinal upset, headache, swelling, and depression are experienced in many contexts. Rather than attending to the features of a particular context, individuals evoke typifications to explain away common symptoms. For instance, one might explain headache as resulting from a lack of sleep, gastrointestinal upset as stemming from overeating, and swelling in the feet as caused by changes in the weather. Throughout my accounts, I displayed doubt that my general symptoms could be tied to Sally's pains. The idea of a sympathetic connection occurred to me only when I experienced unfamiliar or rarely felt bodily sensations.

> About three weeks from term, I experienced a severe migraine. It started above and behind my right temporal lobe, and traveled toward the back of my head. I had further wave-like attacks during dinner and en route to our weekly doctor's appointment. During the day, I had also felt weak, and was experiencing pain in the upper, front thigh area of my left leg. When standing, I thought my leg might collapse.

I did not view the experience of a particular migraine as sympathetic, but I did deem the localized sensation of weakness in one leg, which accompanied the migraine, as suggestive. It was not the headache that suggested the possibility of a sympathetic link, but rather Sally's remark that she had felt pressure and a pinching effect on her uterus and lower abdomen. She thought the baby might be pinching a nerve, since it felt like her right leg was going to collapse. On that same day, I had a similar sensation in my left leg.

Data Excerpt #3

A common element to the experiences highlighted above was my recognition that sympathetic connections always involved unfamiliar or infrequently felt physical sensations that violated my habituated bodily patterns. One of my most surprising connections occurred a few days after our son Nathan was born. I experienced a powerful, unanticipated feeling of increased breast firmness:

> Once breast-feeding began, Sally mentioned how much she liked the tingling sensation, and how her breasts have been firming and hardening since nursing began. Long before her pregnancy and throughout, I have been worried about my breast flabbiness, and my failure to exercise to improve. But I sensed my breasts as firmer during a shower before leaving for the hospital. Upon return, I verified in a mirror that my breasts, which felt firmer, did look harder. I end this entry thus: "My God, that's incredible!"

Research has shown that most men do not recognize possible connections between their symptoms and those of their pregnant partners. Emphasizing the inclusion of men's experiences in maternity nursing, Clinton (1986, 1987) expressed the need for further education and awareness of this phenomenon among expectant fathers. Moreover, early observations by Lipkin and Lamb (1982) showed that medical personnel were also unaware of the phenomenon.

Let's examine what the scholarly research literature has shown. This entails moving from phenomenological descriptive accounts of an unnamed phenomenon to empirical studies that have labeled and named the experience.

SEARCHING FOR MEANING: TURNING TO SCHOLARSHIP FOR CLUES

A systematic search through published research studies drew us to anthropological and cross-cultural research, psychological and psychopathological literatures, and eventually nursing and healthcare studies. It's relevant to follow the research trail in the order outlined, since a critical scholarly attitude reveals how the understanding in one area of inquiry is eventually superseded by another. The sympathetic connections between a pregnant woman and her male partner revolve around the named conception called *couvade*.

There is anthropological research evidence that some men experience sympathetic symptoms similar to the pains experienced by women during pregnancy and labor. The deliberate acting out of pains in sympathy with a pregnant woman is referred to as *ritual couvade*, "a ritual pretence of childbirth" common to many non-Western societies (Trethowan and Conlon, 1965, 57). For example, some fathers have imitated labor pains, some have taken to their beds immediately after the birth and acted like women in confinement, and others have been subjected to strict weight-maintenance diets both during pregnancy and immediately after the birth (58). Explanations for ritual couvade have included such things as a way to ward off evil spirits or redirect male aggression, or simply as something for the male to do. While the magico-religious significance varies from culture to culture, ritual couvade has provided a socially acceptable way for men to participate in the reproductive process.

Ritual couvade, being imitative or simulative, must be distinguished from *couvade syndrome*, wherein the father apparently falls ill (Kupferer, 1965, 101). While ritual couvade refers to "those taboos and practices observed by the father at childbirth," couvade syndrome refers to "the presentation of various physical symptoms that occur in the husbands of pregnant women" (Fishbein, 1981, 356). Below, we emphasize and report on studies on couvade syndrome, since this is the direction of empirical evidence for the phenomenon of sympathetic connections.

PSYCHOPATHOLOGICAL AND PSYCHOLOGICAL EXPLANATIONS FOR COUVADE

Psychological and psychoanalytic theories have been influential in early efforts to explain couvade syndrome scientifically. In the 1930s, Reik was one of the first to offer an interpretation of couvade syndrome which recognized that male connections to pregnancy are of psychogenic origin, and that few men were aware of the ties between their own symptoms and those of their pregnant partners (Trethowan and Conlon, 1965, 58–59). While examining men whom physicians had diagnosed as having clinical disorders, Curtis reaffirmed that most men and their referring physicians had not accounted for the possible influence of impending fatherhood. Curtis claimed that many subjects, including even normal expectant fathers, displayed reactivated childhood sexual fantasies, with more serious clinical cases showing "acting out or impulsive behaviour disorders" (1955, 950).

Based on clinical and case-study methods, researchers have proposed a variety of psychological explanations. Jarvis described four men who became disturbed during their wives' pregnancies or after childbirth as reacting to the emergence of unconscious conflicts (1962, as cited in Osofsky, 1982, 214). Cavenar and Weddington examined three men whose symptoms of abdominal pain suggested couvade syndrome. Unable to isolate a physical cause, they concluded that the three men displayed birth envy at a "nonsexual, preoedipal level," and thus treatment required psychiatric hospitalization (1978, 768). Bittman and Zalk concluded from their case studies that denial is a central factor, since sex-role differences do not permit men to acknowledge their stress during pregnancy. Men have no cultural support to justify feelings of depression, loss of appetite, or nervousness during a woman's pregnancy (1978, 6–7). To avoid creating anxiety for women, men tend to deny their symptoms. Such illustrations, drawn from the psychological literature on couvade syndrome, are representative of those approaches that portray expectant fatherhood as a time when one reactivates childhood fantasies, memories, and conflicts (Heinowitz, 1977, 15–16; Osofsky, 1982).

Criticizing the uncontrolled approach of clinical studies that isolate abnormal cases, Trethowan and Conlon demonstrated that expectant fathers are often affected by their wives' pregnancies. Common symptoms included loss of appetite, nausea, vomiting, and toothache (1965, 65). In a follow-up study, Trethowan reaffirmed that symptoms often are tied to the alimentary tract; yet, the range of couvade symptoms is much greater than originally thought (1968). He also reconfirmed previous reports that most men suffer in silence, without consulting a physician, since they do not recognize the possible ties to pregnancy.

Trethowan maintained that psychological concepts such as repression are too feeble and passive to account for couvade syndrome (1965/1968). In his view, the key underlying factor is identification, a powerful defense mechanism that is accompanied by denial of the basic causes for male anxiety (1968, 113). While anxious men suffer from symptoms such as nausea, morning sickness, and perversion of appetite, Trethowan admitted that it is difficult to explain the male-centered discomfort of toothache, one of the most common complaints. In this regard, he theorized that ritual couvade (as sympathetic magic) is co-present with couvade syndrome (as identification). Expectant fathers develop toothache as a magical act to protect the teeth of their pregnant wives from damage. This notion rests upon the old saw "for every child a tooth" (114).

Despite critiques of psychological explanations for couvade syndrome, very recent research continues to link the conception of identification to couvade as a psychiatric problem. Tenyi, Trixler, and Jádi suggested that certain factors—identification with the expectant mother, ambivalence about fatherhood, perceiving the fetus as a rival, latent homosexuality, parturition envy, and defense against aggressive impulses—play a part in the "psychiatric symptoms" of couvade (1996, 264). Yet another factor, *double identification*, may be responsible for the development of *psychotic couvade*, a rare disorder. Unfortunately, like similar past studies, such claims are based upon a limited, two-case study.

VIEWING COUVADE AS NORMATIVE: CHALLENGING PSYCHOANALYTICAL EXPLANATIONS

Other avenues of inquiry have challenged the notion that couvade is something pathological or problematic. Studies that have documented the incidence of occurrence of couvade syndrome claim that the increasing presence points to a phenomenon that is normative, not psychopathological. Fishbein (1981) and Clinton (1985) established the incidence of occurrence at about 20 percent (reports in the 1960s ranged from 11 to 41 percent). These studies also reaffirm earlier conclusions that most men who seek medical treatment are unaware (as were earlier cohorts) of possible ties to the pregnancy process. Therefore, the reported incidence of couvade syndrome underestimates actual rates of occurrence.

As early as the 1950s, studies reported expectant fathers with symptoms such as abdominal pain, loss of appetite, indigestion, colic, nausea, vomiting, swollen abdomen, weight gain, backache, cramps, depression, and toothache (Curtis, 1955; Trethowan, 1968; Trethowan and Conlon, 1965). Subsequently, Lipkin and Lamb conducted a controlled epidemiologic study of men who sought medical care (during their wives' pregnancies) for couvade-like symptoms that had no other objective explanation (1982). In a similar vein, Bogren interviewed prospective parents to distinguish between male symptoms that occurred during, as opposed to before or after, the pregnancy (1983). And Clinton launched a comprehensive study into the physical and emotional experiences associated with expectant fatherhood (1985).

In rejecting psychoanalytic explanations that treat couvade syndrome as pathology and illness, Clinton approached *modern couvade*[1] as a persistent cultural phenomenon that should be viewed within a nursing-healthcare frame of reference. Unlike the early work on ritual couvade, which explored the pro-social features of this phenomenon relative to specific cultures, research into couvade syndrome has been dominated by psychoanalytic theory. Consequently, researchers approached couvade syndrome as a deviant phenomenon exhibited by neurotic individuals within Western societies (1985, 222–223). Because previous studies relied extensively on the case method and secondhand information (from physicians and family members), research into modern couvade has neglected the "relationship of couvade syndrome to discomforts experienced by the pregnant mate" (225).

Cumulatively, the pioneering work of Lipkin and Lamb (1982), Bogren (1983), and Clinton (1985) identified the most common sympathetic symptoms as gastrointestinal symptoms (abdominal pain, bloating, swelling, cramps), weight changes (usually unintentional gain), changes in appetite, and toothache. Other frequently reported symptoms include nausea, vomiting, leg cramps, backache, fatigue (lassitude), faintness (syncope), irritability (colic), insomnia, and depression (sometimes severe). Clinton also noted additional characteristics such as concern with skin lesions, growths, cysts, sties, sensory organ changes, general feelings of ill health, generalized anxiety, and concern over altered body image (224).

THE EXPANDING EMPIRICAL BASE:
DIRECTIVES FOR THE PHENOMENOLOGICAL PRACTITIONER

Fueled by this increasing body of empirical evidence, researchers began to develop checklists and inventories to track the experience of men and their pregnant partners. Utilizing the commonly reported symptoms of couvade, researchers began developing inventories as the method for learning more about couvade (Black, Holditch-Davis, Sandelowski, and Harris, 1995; Clinton, 1986; Clinton, 1987; Holditch-Davis, Black, Harris, Sandelowski, and Edwards, 1994; Strickland, 1986). The following section outlines how this line of research activity, which accelerated after 1985, has further established the empirical base but done little to expand our understanding of what constitutes the essence of the phenomenon.

Comparative Symptomatology: Building Checklists and Inventories

Clinton used a list of symptoms to determine the presence of couvade in expectant fathers, showing that an overwhelming majority reported at least one symptom during a typical month of their mates' pregnancies (1986). Whether the reporting of a single symptom is parallel to the experience of couvade is unclear. Since many symptoms on the list (for example, headache, nausea, and indigestion) are prevalent in the general population, one would question the comparability. And few differences in the physical symptoms of expectant fathers and nonexpectant controls emerged in a follow-up study (1987).

The *incidence* of couvade symptoms across trimesters depicted by Clinton did not follow the U-shaped pattern (higher incidence of symptoms in the first and third trimesters compared to a drop in symptoms during the second trimester; 1986) that had been reported earlier (Curtis, 1955; Lipkin and Lamb, 1982). Alternately, Strickland found the percentage of expectant fathers experiencing couvade symptoms to be highest during the third trimester, lowest during the first, and in the middle at the second trimester (1986). Similar to Black, et al. (1995), and Holditch-Davis, et al. (1994), Clinton (1986) had difficulty recruiting expectant fathers during the first two months of their mates' pregnancies. In view of the time lag between conception and knowledge of a pregnancy, reports of first-trimester experiences may be underestimated (Patterson, Freese, and Goldenberg, 1986, as cited in Sandelowski and Black, 1994, 604). It is noteworthy, however, that the incidence of couvade syndrome was reported as 34.8 percent of 141 partners of pregnant women at week ten, that is, during their first trimester (Thomas and Upton, 2000). In that study, the syndrome was considered present if two or more symptoms from an itemized list were reported.

In addition to the incidence of couvade symptoms, Clinton had expectant fathers rate the perceived seriousness of each symptom on a Likert scale from 0 (not at all serious) to 10 (very serious). It is noteworthy that a U-shape curve across trimesters did emerge on mean seriousness scores, suggesting that seriousness of expectant fathers' symptoms may be clouding reports of their incidence. During postpartum, expectant fathers reported an average of 7.1 couvade symptoms per month at a seriousness rating of 17.6 (1986, 292–93). That finding, coupled with a subsequent report (1987) that the difference between expectant and nonexpectant fathers in average number, duration, and seriousness of couvade symptoms was greatest during the postpartum period, underscores the importance of the postpartum period in understanding couvade.

To examine the degree of shared pregnancy symptoms, Holditch-Davis, et al., had thirty-six couples with a history of infertility complete the Symptomatology Inventory each month during their pregnancy. Results indicated that six couples may have been manifesting couvade syndrome since they independently reported exact agreement on symptoms more than half the time. Other features of couvade include an intense identification and attunement with a wife who has many symptoms during pregnancy (1994, 546). Since the symptoms were often similar rather than identical, they suggested the term *symptom attunement* to describe the phenomenon. Using the same inventory of symptoms, Black, et al., compared pregnancy symptoms of twenty-one couples with a history of infertility with twelve couples who had no such history. Their results indicated that couples with an infertility history and fertile couples are more alike than different in their reports of pregnancy symptoms. Women have more symptoms than men regardless of fertility status (1995, 6).

Although a heightened awareness of couvade is a consequence of the research reported above, Clinton's (1987) and Klein's (1991) earlier conclusion persists: The phenomenon itself is not well understood. The range of findings from the studies is, no doubt, a reflection of the variation in the criteria, methods, and sampling for couvade (Klein, 1991). For example, the criteria for couvade spanned the reporting of a single symptom in a male partner to agreement about identical or similar symptoms between partners. Previously reported across three trimesters of pregnancy, couvade symptoms emerged during the postpartum period. The number of items on instruments measuring couvade ranged from thirty-two to forty-two. Some symptoms were identical; others, such as bloating/stomach swelling, skin breakdown/sores, were similar; still others (for example, eye problems, increased sexual interest), appeared on only one instrument. The unresolved question, of whether couvade is a male or couple experience, is evident from the different samples used in the research. As Strickland so aptly remarked, without a full account of the syndrome, variances across studies will persist, and the exact incidence of the syndrome in Western society will remain unknown (1986).

Despite many recent, in-depth explorations of couvade symptoms, no clear and consistent pattern has emerged. In an effort to push the knowledge base further, some thinkers have proposed that a conceptual clarification is needed, one that changes the theoretical orientation for undertaking research.

From Empathy to Compathy: Reconceptualizing the Evidence

Couvade experience arises in men's relationships with their pregnant partners: no pregnancy, no syndrome; no partner, no pregnancy. That fact influenced Black, et al. (1995), and Holditch-Davis, et al. (1994), to focus on couple's experience of couvade. The focus on couples is consistent with Morse and Mitcham's conceptualization of *compathy* to account for couvade. They defined *compathy* as the acquisition of the distress and/or physiological symptoms (including pain) of others by an apparently healthy individual following contact with the physical distress of another (1997, 650). They stated further that *compathetic contagion* is especially strong when there is a close relationship with the person in distress, an obvious occurrence in the pregnant couple.

The *compathetic response*, which is evoked by the experiences of another, can be manifest, suppressed, or blocked (Morse and Mitcham, 1997). It is a manifest response that is evident in the reporting of couvade symptoms by expectant fathers. An expectant father's manifest response may be similar or dissimilar to that of his partner. Morse and Mitcham identified (a) a similar response that is less intense as *initiated*, (b) one that is similar and has the same intensity as *identical*, and (c) one that is similar but worse or exaggerated as *transferred*. This conceptualization is consistent with Holditch-Davis, et al., who reported that couvade symptoms between pregnant partners can be similar (1994).

Clinton examined the seriousness of symptoms reported by expectant fathers; however, her focus on men's instead of couples' experience of couvade does not provide evidence for compathy (1986). Other studies, such as research by Storey, Walsh, Quinton, and Wynne-Edwards, indicate that hormone levels of pregnant partners are also related. Using blood samples, normally drawn at one of four points before and after the child's birth, they examined the relationship between hormone levels and paternal responsiveness in thirty-four Canadian couples. The strongest correlation reported was between men's blood hormone levels and those of their pregnant partners, a finding interpreted as a link between communication within the couple and physiological responses in men (2000, 11).

Not surprisingly, genetic and medical scientists have entered this research arena and partnered with psychologists, thus resurrecting an explanatory schema that nursing-based researchers had begun to question. These investigations have focused on relationships between biological factors and symptoms, including emotional responses. For example, Storey, et al. (2000), reported that male partners of pregnant women who reported at least two couvade symptoms had higher blood prolactin levels than those with no symptoms; and those with lower blood testosterone during the postpartum period demonstrated more nurturing behaviors. Further, Berg and Wynne-Edwards confirmed that men's prolactin levels increased and testosterone levels decreased as their wives approached childbirth (2001). Their results were based on saliva samples of twenty-three men recruited during first-trimester prenatal classes and followed until three months postpartum.

What, then, has the array of empirical investigations, as reviewed above, done to expand our understanding of the phenomenon of sympathetic connections between a pregnant woman and her male partner? We know more about the incidence, about the variety of possible symptomatic connections, and about physiological correlates between a man and his pregnant partner. Yet, we know nothing more about the *whatness* of the phenomenon, something that phenomenological inquiry offers as distinct from, yet related to, the insights from empirical human science inquiry. We are drawn to question the utility of spending additional resources (financial and human) to continue the large-scale inventory trail. Like the dilemma posed by Ockham's razor, what's the point of undertaking yet one more large-scale inventory study to fine-tune what is already overly finely tuned?

REVISITING THE UTILITY OF PHENOMENOLOGY: UNCOVERING TACIT ASSUMPTIONS UNDERLYING EMPIRICAL STUDIES

Contrary to widespread misconception, phenomenology was never generated as an alternative to the empirical sciences. As a foundational enterprise, Edmund Husserl sought to provide the philosophical basis upon which the empirical sciences could be constituted on "solid ground." Husserl's work sought (a) to found philosophy phenomenologically, serving as the basis of all science, and (b) to generate a phenomenological psychology upon which an empirical psychology could be erected. In this section, we display how the limits of empirical studies serve as an invitation to further phenomenological exploration.

Clinton's switch from *couvade syndrome* to *modern couvade* seemed to herald a shift in thinking away from pathology and deviance toward health and normalcy (1985). The progressive establishment of the frequency of couvade symptoms reinforces the necessity and inevitability of the switch. The change in name alone, however, has been insufficient to advance our understanding of the phenomenon. Even though conceptual and methodological emphasis is given to couvade symptoms, many researchers revert to the use of *couvade syndrome* when discussing study results. Moreover, it is unlikely that further empirical specification will provide insight into the essential nature of this intersubjective experience.

The checklist approach is problematic on several counts: (a) its use is restrictive since it delimits the experiences, thus additions, deletions, or modifications to the symptom list are precluded; and (b) the approach may also be alerting men to find connections which may well be groundless or tied to other medical and bodily conditions. While inventories and checklists have served to document further the incidence of occurrence, they do not provide deeper access to the nature of couvade as a phenomenon.

Neither will conceptual substitution, such as that available in Morse and Mitcham's concept of compathy (1997), get at the *whatness* of this phenomenon. Nonetheless, the concept does shift thinking from a male's to a couples' experience, and highlights the relevance of studying qualifiers such as intensity. It is not the concept itself, however, but an unpackaging of the meaning of such conceptions that can help us understand what couvade is. In this vein, research approaches such as phenomenology treat conceptions such as compathy as openings to in-depth inquiry rather than as explanatory closings.

While ideas like compathy have extended our knowledge of the range and types of sympathetic symptoms, there is still little understanding as to why few men recognize the possible link between their symptoms and those experienced by their pregnant partners. In this regard, a phenomenological approach can help one identify sympathetic connections. Clinton's initial proposal for a comprehensive study of modern couvade had an implicit phenomenological component whereby the emotional and physical experiences of individual men would find expression and social validation (1985, 234). Yet, the direction taken by Clinton and others after 1985 never developed the analytical potential inherent in in-depth descriptive expressions of individual experience.

TAKING STOCK: COMBINING EMPIRICAL RESULTS WITH PHENOMENOLOGICAL INSIGHTS

The research reviewed in this essay reports on the findings of biopsychosocial investigations of couvade syndrome. The personal account available through one couple's experience of pregnancy and the childbirth process offers a very different portal to understanding the phenomenon. Both perspectives can inform the encounters of healthcare practitioners with pregnant couples. We close with a comment on how scholarship can inform practice, and how we have been transformed by approaching our own research studies phenomenologically.

The scholar-practitioner model is embraced by health professionals whose research questions often originate in practice, with the clinical setting being a rich laboratory wherein theory is tested and research evidence guides praxis (McClintock, 2004). Furthermore, praxis is central to educative activities in the curricula of health professional programs (Bevis and Watson, 1989).

In view of the empirically rich link between couvade symptoms and expectant fatherhood, health professionals should be attending to fathers'

experiences with pregnancy and the childbirth process as integral components of their practice. The scope of fathers' experiences suggests that there
are ample opportunities to include them in anticipatory health teaching
and counseling sessions, such as doctor's visits, prenatal classes, diagnostic
appointments, and home visits. During such encounters, health professionals can provide expectant fathers with information about the relationship between the transition to fatherhood and their emotional status and
physical health (Clinton, 1987). As wise practitioners, health professionals
should also be prepared to move beyond their existing stock of knowledge
to question what they may have taken for granted or overlooked in fathers'
experiences. Their quests for deeper understandings will not only more
fully inform their practices, it will also encourage fathers to explore their
physical and emotional responses to their wives' pregnancy. The lessons in
this essay are a reminder to integrate patients' experiences as part of the evidence that guides the practice of healthcare.

As displayed in this chapter, descriptive experiential accounts can contribute to our understanding of male connections to pregnancy, labor, delivery, and postpartum childbirth. In David Rehorick's experience, such
recognition was enhanced when he attended to unusual sensations and vi-
olations to habituated bodily patterns. In phenomenological terms, this
means attending to lived experience without imposing preconceived categories upon or judging the worthiness of any experience. One seeks to describe the phenomenon as it presents itself.

This attitude contrasts sharply with psychological and psychoanalytic approaches, which have conceptualized couvade syndrome as deviant and
pathological. Doing so isolates and decontextualizes male experiences from
the broader cultural context within which they become meaningful. A turn
to the immediacy of experience is a starting point for a phenomenology of
the body that provides an account of embodiment from the view of the subject (Turner, 1984, 54). Phenomenology, as conceived by Maurice Merleau-
Ponty (1962), never treats the body as a physical object, but, instead, as an
embodiment of a consciousness which is intentional (Turner, 1984, 53 and
59). When the insights of phenomenological discovery are coupled to the
findings of empirical research, our understanding of any phenomenon is
fuller and richer. But meaning making is, first and foremost, a purposive act,
one that is grounded in a phenomenological account of human experience.

PERSONAL TRANSFORMATION:
A CLOSING NOTE FROM LINDA NUGENT

Since the influence of phenomenology on David's life and work has been
explicated in chapter 1, this essay closes with a commentary by Linda about

the relevance of phenomenology and interpretive studies to her life, work, and research in the health and nursing sciences:

Although I, Linda, have returned to empirical work in the health sciences, my time in the world of phenomenology has made me a more thoughtful and reflective empirical researcher. I was introduced to interpretive studies in a doctoral course with David at the University of New Brunswick in Canada. Although eager to learn about different research methodologies, I felt discomfort and anxiety, and doubted my ability to *get it* during the initial classes of the semester.

In David's graduate seminar, I decided to explore my experience as a family caregiver to my dying mother. I began a phenomenological study with six participants to examine the meaning of *family caregiving*. Having done prior research with family caregivers, I was confident that I could understand their world, yet curious enough to wonder if there were additional insights to be gained. By the end of the study, I was challenging my taken-for-granted understandings. In addition, a careful reflection on my own experience as a caregiving daughter allowed me to see that family caregiving, especially as a nurse, got in the way of being a daughter.

Although the term *caregiver* implies a unidirectional relationship, I will never forget and always be grateful to my mother for picking out clothes and selecting the hymns and pallbearers for her funeral, helping write her own obituary, and advising against a wake at home. My mother's gift not only spared the family energy the morning she died, it gave us all comfort in knowing we were doing things right.

Since venturing into the world of phenomenology and interpretive studies, I am more sensitive to openings that people and research participants provide during data collection events, such as interviewing. Rather than viewing such openings as intrusions or distractions (as I had before studying phenomenology), I honestly pursue them. The opportunity to encounter interpretive ways of knowing has had lasting effects on my work and life. Although my career has drawn me away from phenomenological scholarship as an explicit enterprise, I know that my prior work informs the way that I do my career work and the quality of my empirical research projects, some of which are changing the healthcare agenda of government officials and politicians within the province of New Brunswick in eastern Canada.

NOTES

1. It is curious that Clinton's efforts to shift couvade from pathological to normative perspectives entailed a creative relabeling from *couvade syndrome* to *modern couvade*. This removed the negative psychological baggage associated

with the conception of *syndrome*; however, in subsequent research publications, Clinton reverted (without clear explanation) to the earlier notion of *couvade syndrome*.

REFERENCES

Berg, Sandra J., and Katherine E. Wynne-Edwards. (2001) Changes in Testosterone, Cortisol, and Estradiol Levels in Men Becoming Fathers. *Mayo Clinic Proceedings*, 76(6), 582–93.

Bevis, Em O., and Jean Watson. (1989) *Toward a Caring Curriculum: A New Pedagogy for Nursing*. New York: National League of Nursing.

Bittman, Sam, and Sue Rosenberg Zalk. (1978) *Expectant Fathers*. New York: Hawthorn Books.

Black, Beth Perry, Diane Holditch-Davis, Margarete Sandelowski, and B. Glenn Harris. (1995) Comparison of Pregnancy Symptoms of Infertile and Fertile Couples. *Journal of Perinatal & Neonatal Nursing*, 9(2), 1–9.

Bogren, Lennart Y. (1983) Couvade. *Acta Psychiatrica Scandinavica*, 68, 55–65.

Cavenar, Jesse O., Jr., and William W. Weddington, Jr. (1978) Abdominal Pain in Expectant Fathers. *Psychosomatics*, 19(12), 761–68.

Clinton, Jacqueline F. (1985) Couvade: Patterns, Predictors, and Nursing Management: A Research Proposal Submitted to the Division of Nursing. *Western Journal of Nursing Research*, 7(2), 221–43.

———. (1986) Expectant Fathers at Risk for Couvade. *Nursing Research*, 35(6), 290–95.

———. (1987) Physical and Emotional Responses of Expectant Fathers Throughout Pregnancy and the Early Postpartum Period. *International Journal of Nursing Studies*, 24(1), 59–68.

Curtis, James L. (1955) A Psychiatric Study of 55 Expectant Fathers. *U.S. Armed Forces Medical Journal*, 6(7), 937–50.

Fishbein, Eileen Grief. (1981) The Couvade: A Review. *Journal of Gynecological Nursing, September/October*, 356–59.

Heinowitz, Jack R. (1977) *Becoming a Father for the First Time: A Phenomenological Study*. Unpublished Doctoral Dissertation. The California School of Professional Psychology.

Holditch-Davis, Diane, Beth Perry Black, B. Glenn Harris, Margarete Sandelowski, and Lloyd J. Edwards. (1994) Beyond Couvade: Pregnancy Symptoms in Couples with a History of Infertility. *Health Care for Women International*, 15(6), 537–48.

Jarvis, Wilbur. (1962) Some Effects of Pregnancy and Childbirth on Men. *Journal of the American Psychoanalytical Association*, 10(4), 689–700.

Klein, H. (1991) Couvade Syndrome: Male Counterpart to Pregnancy. *International Journal of Psychiatry in Medicine*, 21(1), 57–69.

Kupferer, Harriet J. K. (1965) Couvade: Ritual or Real Illness. *American Anthropologist*, 67 (February), 99–101.

Lipkin, Mack, Jr., and Gerri S. Lamb. (1982) The Couvade Syndrome: An Epidemiologic Study. *Annals of Internal Medicine*, 96(4), 509–11.

McClintock, Charles. (2004) The Scholar-Practitioner Model. In A. DiStefano, K. E. Rudestam, and R. J. Silverman (eds.), *Encyclopedia of Distributed Learning* (393–96). Thousand Oaks, CA: Sage.

Merleau-Ponty, Maurice. (1962) *Phenomenology of Perception* (C. Smith, trans.). London: Routledge & Kegan Paul. (Original work published 1945)

Morse, Janice M., and Carl Mitcham. (1997) Compathy: The Contagion of Physical Distress. *Journal of Advanced Nursing, 26*(4), 649–57.

Osofsky, Howard J. (1982). Expectant and New Fatherhood as a Developmental Crisis. *Bulletin of the Menninger Clinic, 46*(3), 209–30.

Sandelowski, Margarete, and Beth Perry Black. (1994) The Epistemology of Expectant Parenthood. *Western Journal of Nursing Research, 16*(6), 601–22.

Storey, Anne E., Carolyn J. Walsh, Roma L. Quinton, and Katherine E. Wynne-Edwards. (2000) Hormonal Correlates of Paternal Responsiveness in New and Expectant Fathers. *Evolution and Human Behavior, 21*(2), 79–95.

Strickland, Ora L. (1986) The Occurrence of Symptoms in Expectant Fathers. *Nursing Research, 36*(3), 184–89.

Tenyi, Tamas, Matyas Trixler, and Ferenc Jádi. (1996) Psychotic Couvade: 2 Case Reports. *Psychopathology, 29*, 252–54.

Thomas, S. Grace, and Dominic Upton. (2000) Expectant Fathers' Attitudes Towards Pregnancy. *British Journal of Midwifery, 8*(4), 218–21.

Trethowan, William H. (1965) Sympathy Pains. *Discovery, 26*(January), 30–33.

———. (1968) The Couvade Syndrome: Some Further Observations. *Journal of Psychosomatic Research, 12*,107–15.

Trethowan, William H., and M. F. Conlon. (1965) The Couvade Syndrome. *British Journal of Psychiatry, 111*(January), 57–66.

Turner, Bryan S. (1984) *The Body and Society*. Oxford: Basil Blackwell.

3

Experiencing Phenomenology as Mindful Transformation

An Autobiographical Account

Sandra K. Simpson

> Mindful inquiry springs from the lifeworld of the researcher. . . . Within the lifeworld, you may view the entire research process as a journey between yourself and texts—that is, something to be interpreted. (Bentz and Shapiro, 1998, 42)

There is now ample documentation that captures the experience of what individuals face when coming to phenomenology for the first time (for example, see Bentz, 1995; Hultgren, 1995; Rehorick and Taylor, 1995). What is missing is a full account of the transformative nature of coming to, sticking with, and then emerging from deep encounters with phenomenological texts, thinkers, and practice. In this chapter, I report on my own personal experience of encountering the phenomenological and hermeneutic domains of inquiry. My Ph.D. dissertation was a *showing* of this process (Simpson, 2003). This chapter is a reflective *telling* of my story, one that treats the completed dissertation as the phenomenon, a product that displays my sense of *becoming* a phenomenologist. In an abbreviated form, I will reveal features of my self-transformation as a scholar, which, in turn, has changed the way I practice as a professional psychologist. The transformative process emerges through a tacking between extensive and continuing journal accounts of my lived experience and my efforts to grasp the texts of phenomenological thinkers and apply them to my own lifeworld.

DISCOVERING PHENOMENOLOGY AND HERMENEUTICS
AS PHILOSOPHY AND PRACTICE

My work with clients in psychotherapy has been about their difficulty in making life changes, something that I have witnessed again and again. Witnessing their struggle has made me more aware of my own personal issues and concerns. It puzzled me as to why this is so. If we can formulate a plan to make change and seem to know what we want and need to do, why do we hesitate and often refuse to take steps toward change?

As I was working with such issues, I discovered hermeneutic phenomenology, found myself intrigued, and began to think that becoming a phenomenologist might very well facilitate the types of change that I was interested in studying. I was inspired by Bentz and Shapiro's presentation of a foundation and perspective from which to engage in the research process.

> We have seen how one's research can contribute to the transformation of one's self or identity. We have experienced this ourselves and seen it in our students. We are always noticing how values shape conceptual frameworks, and we believe that research needs to be thought of in connection with all of the ways that it is part of individuals' lives and lifeworlds. . . . We strongly believe that your awareness of and reflection on your world, and the intellectual awareness and reflection that are woven into your research, affect—or should affect—one another. (1998, 5)

I set for myself the task of becoming a hermeneutic phenomenologist. In order to do this, I read extensively about both phenomenology and hermeneutics. It was necessary to learn about these traditions before I could understand what it means to link them together. I learned from teachers, colleagues who were working on similar projects, and other scholars who have written about both traditions. I created a reading pathway into the writings and practice of selected phenomenological scholars. The mindmap in Figure 3.1 displays my point of departure.

I came to realize that it is possible to read, learn, and think about phenomenology without yet being a phenomenologist. The *being* of phenomenology involves specific activities to bring oneself into a place where a deep involvement with a phenomenon can occur. Phenomenological scholars often make the point that phenomenology requires a "radically different way of being" (Bentz, 1995, 60). Francine Hultgren quotes one of her students: "Phenomenology is not simply learning a research method, it is truly a 'way of being,' a philosophy of life" (1995, 379). This brings us, again, to the challenge of balancing

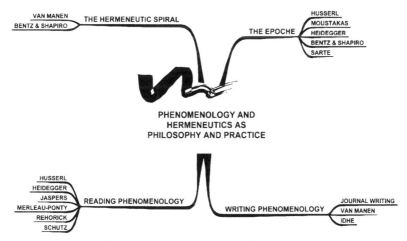

Figure 3.1. Phenomenology and Hermeneutics as Philosophy and Practice

the learning, the practice, and the research involved in becoming a phenomenologist.

My Practice

The term *practice* implies a process that contains some structure and indicates how work gets done. It also refers to doing something in order to get better at it, such as practicing a musical instrument or playing a sport. To begin my practice of hermeneutic phenomenology, I had to identify the phenomenon to be studied. The phenomenon became *understanding what phenomenology is about.* My reading suggested that three concepts were central to this goal: exploring becoming a phenomenologist, being mindful, and understanding transformation. Max van Manen's words were helpful to me:

> For all phenomenological research, in all its stages, [it] is [necessary] to be constantly mindful of one's original question and thus to be steadfastly oriented to the lived experience that makes it possible to ask the "what it is like" question in the first place. (1990, 42)

The Hermeneutic Spiral: A Compelling Conception

A particularly compelling concept in hermeneutics is that of the *hermeneutic spiral*, referring to a spiral of encountering a phenomenon, and then working to describe, interpret, and understand the phenomenon (see Bentz, 1989; Bentz and Shapiro, 1998). We may begin with a question or a concept that guides our explorations. As we seek understanding, we travel a spiral that brings us close to understanding as the spiral tightens. When we reach an initial understanding, the spiral opens up once again, with this initial understanding pointing to a question or concept.

Another way to think about the spiral is as a manifold or strata of interpretation, with each layer taking us into a deeper and richer place of awareness and knowledge. The understanding reached at each layer suggests the way into the next layer, as we continue to explore the depths of understanding that can be achieved. While practicing hermeneutic phenomenology, it is necessary to have patience and a willingness to not fully understand the meaning in the beginning. It is necessary to remain open and curious, and to trust that understanding will come.

Reading Phenomenology: Grasping at Bits of Text

Reading phenomenology is another step in the practice of hermeneutic phenomenology. The early work in phenomenology was written in German and French, and reading in translation is sometimes problematic. I first began to learn about phenomenology from presentations and research workshops. It was both intriguing and difficult to understand. The intrigue came from the idea that it was an experiential process that incorporates the consciousness and deep engagement of the student. My work in gestalt and existential psychology prepared me to be receptive to this idea. My natural way of being in the world is compatible with phenomenology, as I have learned over the past years of my work. The difficulty is similar to the difficulty encountered in learning any new philosophy. There is the need to learn a new *language*, in the sense of a nomenclature, pointing to new ways of thinking about what we may think we already know.

As I began to dip into the reading of the early European phenomenologists, I realized that I would read phenomenological philosophy, write about it, and practice it without ever coming to grasp it fully. This is part of its wonder and fascination for me. Phenomenology is mysterious. It appeals to my sense of pleasure in discovery as I continue to catch glimmers of meaning. I am in phenomenology's grasp as surely as I am human. At some deep, and yet unknown, level, I must continue to work, as Heidegger suggests, to *see phenomenologically* (1962). This work will never be finished.

Reading phenomenology is a challenge essential to understanding and becoming a phenomenologist. Getting a taste, a bit of flavor for it, is necessary but not sufficient to this becoming. It must be studied, puzzled over, and not taken at face value. I read phenomenology with my intellect, my heart, and my body. It turned into an intense engagement with writers such as Husserl (1965), Heidegger (1962), Jaspers (1994), and many more.

WRITING AND PHENOMENOLOGY:
THE USE OF MY JOURNALS

Van Manen suggests that "to do research in a phenomenological sense is already and immediately and always a bringing to speech of something. And this thoughtfully bringing to speech is most commonly a writing activity" (1990, 32). This was particularly relevant to my study and the way I continue to practice hermeneutic phenomenology. He suggests that writing and research is a "poetizing activity" (13) as well as a search for what it means to be human: "to construct a possible interpretation of the nature of a certain human experience" (41). As I read van Manen closely, I began to see that "a certain human experience" that I wanted to understand is the human experience of transformation. I began to wonder about the extent to which my twenty years of journal writing might be inherently phenomenological in nature.

Alfred Schutz discusses in some detail the phenomenology of meaning. He says that humans cannot understand themselves in the moment, the immediacy of their experience. He suggests that we can only know ourselves in retrospect. He also suggests that it is important that we know ourselves

> in the entire range of [our] own . . . experiences. . . . Here and here only, in the deepest stratum of experience that is accessible to reflection, is to be found the ultimate source of the phenomena of "meaning" and "understanding." This stratum of experience can only be disclosed in strictly philosophical self-consciousness. (1967, 12)

Journal writing has been an essential and continuing practice for me. I have written from an existential stream of consciousness to bring to light and have before me the activity of my intellect, my emotions, and my consciousness for the purpose of better understanding myself—to have text from my deep consciousness to interpret, to uncover what is hidden beneath the everydayness of my thought, and to seek to understand the meaning of my being in the world.

In her book, *Becoming Mature: Childhood Ghosts and Spirits in Mature Life*, Bentz (1989, 1) presents a grounded theory of adult development, one approached through an application of hermeneutic phenomenology. Bentz uses extensive data that she collected in the process of her research with fifty-three women as she explored how childhood experiences shape the lives of adults. Two sources of data from her participants were written autobiographies and present-time journal writing. It was significant to my work that the use of these research methods was found to be transformational for both the participants who produced the written material and the researcher who interpreted it.

As I studied this research, I came to see how the extensive collection of journal writing that I had produced over a twenty-year period could be a rich source of data for my own personal quest. My journal writing provided me with a way to make the personal experience of my self-consciousness accessible for reflection.

The data for my explorations involved returning to approximately fifteen hundred to two thousand pages of written text generated over two decades. The decision to study my personal lifeworld was not made lightly, nor was it easy to do. I was concerned about charges of self-indulgence, and becoming lost within my own stories. Treated as a research project, Bentz and Shapiro characterize the process as "a journey between myself and [the] texts" (1998, 42) of my lived experience of personal transformation, learning the ever-challenging way of mindfulness, and learning to be a phenomenologist.

In the end, there were several compelling reasons for studying myself. First, I had data; it was readily available, and there was lots of it. Second, I'm comfortable in first learning from myself, and then moving out to learn from and teach others. Third, the phenomenological scholars who were mentoring me encouraged this turn. As my research unfolded, I continued journaling, as always, but I added a new component: writing about my experience of trying to understand phenomenology.

As I experimented with the hermeneutic spiral of interpretation, core concepts emerged in interpreting the journal texts. These concepts can be described as phenomenological tools of interpretation, and they are my core discoveries:

- *Themes*: Meaningful life themes emerged during the interpretation of the journal writing.
- *Identity moments*: During the analysis of the data, I began to see specific entries that were transformational at the moment of analysis.
- *Paradoxes*: Numerous paradoxes appeared in my journal writing, and highlighting these was enlightening and deepened my self-awareness.
- *Meditation koans*: As I noticed the paradoxes appearing, I began to see that they had elements of Zen koans, enigmatic sayings often used by Zen Buddhist masters as objects for teaching through meditation.

Each of these core concepts contained an array of elements that emerged from an in-depth analysis of my journals. Figure 3.2 depicts these elements.

The elements surfaced through successive interpretive turns, which Bentz and Shapiro express this way:

> We visualize the journey of the research process as a spiral to emphasize the sense of expansion and forward motion that comes from circling in time and

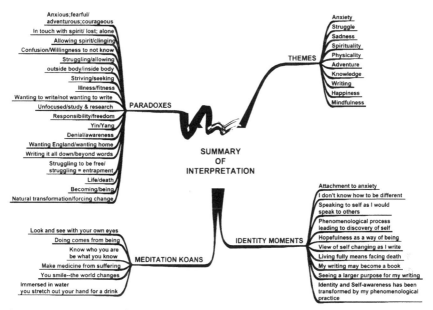

Figure 3.2.   Summary of Interpretation

touching various points, each time from a new point in time and in one's own self-development. (1998, 42)

I experienced the spiral of the research process as a series of turns, "mediated by an empty space on the spiral, indicating that [I was] moving through lived time and . . . living through the meaning of this new aspect of becoming a mindful inquirer" (43). Each turn in the spiral represented different aspects of the research process and each space between the turns in the spiral was experienced as a pause in the work. I found these spaces between turns to occur naturally and necessarily. It was necessary to pause and allow the practices of my work to settle into thoughts and feelings about what was happening.

The spiral began with the gathering together of all the pages of my journal writing. I had not written every day during those twenty years; however, I wrote extensively within each year and I always wrote when I was trying to understand some aspect of my lived experience. Once I began to look deeply at the texts of my life's experience, there would never again be a time when I wouldn't *see* myself in a new way. I had to ask myself if this was something I really wanted to do. Did I want to see myself in new, possibly unexpected, ways? Was I willing to allow others to see as well? I resolved to move rather quickly into the texts before such questions barred me from any movement at all.

I started by reading through the journals from beginning to end. My initial reading was to get a sense of what I had written about and determine which journals, from which time periods, I would choose to interpret. The first reading was surprising in some ways and sobering in others. I was surprised by depth of the writing, my continued dedication to the task, and the relevance of the material to the phenomenological quest at hand. Clearly, there was sufficient and appropriate data for the study. I was sobered by the recurrent expressions of painful and difficult aspects of my life, rather than the beauty, opportunities, and blessings.

This turn in the hermeneutic spiral of interpretation was slow as I read and allowed what was there to emerge. I approached this reading meditatively. I just read, took no notes, and allowed myself to be immersed in my own words. I approached the work as if I knew nothing about it and harbored no preconceptions. In subsequent readings, I began the next step, which entailed looking for themes and patterns, deciding how to organize what appeared, and returning to the research literatures that were informing my study and my methodology.

In the next turn, I chose the chunks of writing from the journals that would be the data to be interpreted. I noticed that my writing changed at a particular point in time from a sort of diary or report of daily life to an exploration of my lived experience. So I chose to begin at that shift. I read and highlighted words and phrases that caught my attention and seemed meaningful, even if I didn't know why. At first, this process seemed chaotic and not scholarly. As I sensed that themes were emerging, I felt reassured and my study deepened. As I continued to seek themes, I recognized that there were other organizing conceptions that I came to call paradoxes, identity moments, and meditation koans.

This stage of the exploration was not as emotionally charged as the early, beginning work. I was able to step away from the emotional content and I became fascinated by what I was seeing. However, at this point, it was as if the data came from someone other than me. I made some comments about the identity moments, paradoxes, and meditation koans in my data analysis scheme, as relevant ideas surfaced during my explorations. Multiple rereadings of the journals engendered a comfortable relationship with the texts.

The next step in the process was to group the words and phrases that I had recorded into meaningful themes. Two themes surfaced in a clear and strong way; others surprised me. Following is only a sample of the kinds of thematic patterns that surfaced from my journal logs.

Theme: Anxiety
What I want to do is drop deeply inside myself and understand more about my anxiousness and avoidance. I am so afraid. I am afraid to be my full self.

While I can explain this away with a psychological interpretation, I cannot seem to really know what it is that I fear so much. But—I do believe this feeling is fear. I believe with all my mind that I want to experience my whole self. Yet, I fight it. Why? . . . Perhaps I am not meant to break free of it . . . perhaps, it is my life task to move beyond it by remembering the pain and the price one pays for not pushing through the fear. Not to ever truly be rid of the fear, but to act impeccably in spite of it.

This is the theme that I noticed early in the reading of my journals. I soon began to see how attached I was to being anxious and fearful. I was shocked to see how I describe myself again and again, day after day, year after year, as an anxious, fearful, phobic person.

There was a moment, during this turn of the analysis, when my awareness of my attachment to anxiety as a way of being became an identity moment for me. This was both a stunning and sad realization. Yet there was also a quick glimmer of hope. In the beginning of this realization, I allowed myself time to experience strong feelings of sadness, regret, and loss. These were not feelings of self-pity but feelings of self-empathy. Pity is a feeling that includes judging a person, or oneself, as pitiful, perhaps weak, and unable to care for herself. Empathy conveys a sense of understanding and being with a person, or oneself, in a nonjudgmental, accepting way. This was an interesting and meaningful learning, and an example of mindful transformation.

BEYOND THEMES: EMERGENT INSIGHTS

As I was first reading my journals and identifying themes, I noticed the ways in which I wrote about such issues as anxiety, struggling, and sadness. Again, I was keyed in to the ways in which I saw myself in a psychologically negative or neurotic way. I experienced myself as flawed and troubled. As I continued to go back into the writing, using a hermeneutic phenomenological approach, I began to see that I also wrote about being happy, spiritual, adventuresome, and mindful. It is striking to me that it was the meditative, phenomenological process that allowed me to discover this. This was another identity moment.

As I looked at the themes as they emerged, I was struck by the order in which I chose to articulate them. There is, in a psychological sense, an evolutionary quality to the emergence of my awareness of the themes. I also see this evolution as another hermeneutic spiraling process. At the beginning of the spiral is the presenting of a psychological problem. In this case, the initial problem would be seen as anxiety. Anxiety often presents as a struggle with the self. Once this is seen and acknowledged, other feelings are then noticed and experienced. This is the second turn of the spiral, and sadness was the next feeling to emerge. As I studied it, I wrote that I was actually encouraged that I was able to identify the feeling of sadness as I wrote and reviewed my journals. In a psychological sense, the awareness of feeling sad is seen as progress.

The next themes that I saw were spirituality and physicality, which emerged during the third turn in the spiral. I was moving out of the anxiety, struggle, and sadness to an awareness of myself as a spiritual and physical being. This is a view of being that has a gestalt quality—seeing myself more holistically. At this point, I began to see other qualities of my life that are less introverted. In yet another turn of the spiral, I began to recognize the happiness in my life and the activities that I cherish and aspire to: adventure, being a writer, and seeking knowledge. Finally, I became aware of the quality of mindfulness that permeates my journals. This awareness brings me full circle, preparing me for whatever the next level of insight and inspiration might bring.

Paradoxes Within the Themes

As I have explored my own psychology and been a companion to others exploring their life issues, I have been aware of the struggles we often experience with different aspects of our being. We juxtapose our personal qualities as *either/or*; we split off qualities that we believe are somehow not good, and seek to maintain those qualities that we can accept and admire. One of my discoveries in this study was the reality and the acceptance of paradox within my being. I am both an anxious person and an adventurous, courageous person. I like to see myself as a writer, yet I resist and struggle with writing. I accuse myself of being unfocused and scattered, although I have completed several academic degrees. There were many examples of paradoxes within the themes of my life. To see these ways of being and accept them, fully, was transformational for me. Here is one illustration of paradox within my writings:

Paradox: "I am not becoming, I am" (Pablo Picasso, exact source unknown)
I understand this paradox in this way. The truth of my Being is with me always. It is obscured by many things and the way to reach my truth is the phenomenological and Buddhist way.

These two ways are the same for me: the Epoche is the space I clear when I enter into meditation. It is in the Epoche that I can see and begin my journey inward toward my True Self, my Being. However, I cannot command or demand from this place. I have to wait. Quietly, patiently. I have to trust that what I need to see and understand will show itself. It is this process that has been the blockage for me.

In my heart, I knew this truth, but I did not trust my heart. I believed (in my head) that I had to do something else of an intellectual nature to accomplish what I wanted my [study] to be. The Epoche, the meditative state, seems too spiritual to be appropriate for writing a research project. Yet, my topic chose me and there is no other way to approach this topic but through the Epoche, the place of meditation [Another paradox].

What can be done? There is only one thing that can be done. Experience and describe this state of Being first—and then write about the journey that brought me here. This is the hermeneutics of the work—because I know that each time I describe the process, the state of being that I began from will shift and become richer, deeper, more true, better understood. So beginning at the end is not really beginning at the end, because the "end" will change, transform, each time I approach it. And so, I have begun, again, and the beginning is the end, again.

So, transformation is also a paradox—between becoming and already being. It is necessary to sit in the tension, to accept that both are truthful and meaningful. It is in this tension that I will learn something of what I want to know, that I will find out more about that voice within me that already knows and can speak if I will listen.

I can see now that this is not a small voice at all, just a quiet one. This voice doesn't shout, it's calm, and sure and waiting, knowing that her time is close when she will be fully heard, acknowledged, allowed. This voice has the wisdom of my intuition.

Meditation Koans

As I was exploring the theme of spirituality, I began to observe meaning emerging that had the quality of meditation koans. The idea of the koan comes from Zen Buddhism. Koans are insightful sayings used by Zen teachers as a focus of meditation practice that can lead the practitioner to wisdom. Several koans appeared during the discovery of themes. I share one as a demonstration of how mindfulness and hermeneutic phenomenology opened me to meaning and insightfulness.

A Zen koan: Immersed in water, you stretch out your hands for a drink
I am in the midst of exactly what I have asked for in my life. I have time for writing; I have a safe and secure place to do it. I even know what I want to write about and have a plan for writing it. Immersed in water, I reach out my hand for a drink. Why am I afraid? Of what? Of being seen, of someone knowing what is in my heart and at the depths of my soul, for it is only from my heart and my soul that I can write. Can I trust those who will read my writing to know this? Can I allow who I am, what I believe, to be seen by others? Immersed in water, I reach out my hand for a drink.

As I write this I become quivery inside; a small voice quivers within. Can I listen? Can I allow this voice to speak, and promise that fearful little soul a safe space, in time and place, to be herself? For this is at the root of my transformation, of my becoming. Immersed in water, I reach out my hand for a drink.

In truth, I am not really becoming, I already am. Transformation for me is not somehow changing my outer self, or, for that matter, my inner self. It is allowing myself to experience the truth of who I am, who have I always been, and yet have been afraid to be.

Identity Moments: Becoming a Phenomenologist

I have noted several instances of identity moments as I have told this story. These moments shifted my personal sense of self and were transformational. I include one more, since it reflects who I see as the person that I now am:

> What does it mean to be a writer, scholar, teacher? Meaning is what phenomenology seeks to uncover. Meaning is what is found from an interpretation of experience . . . from the Epoche. So, I have to be these things before I can truly know what this means.
>
> I write, I teach, I engage in scholarly philosophical reading, interpretation, writing, discussing, dialoguing, pondering. So, I am a scholar, writer, teacher. Why is this so difficult to own? Ownership can be quiet and still and humble. I can be just what I am—no fanfare, no self-aggrandizing—just being. This is who I am. It isn't a job, a role—it just is. I want to own this, to be comfortable with this identity, with this being. Writing, teaching, and scholarship are work. There is no magic—beyond the everyday magic of loving one's work. This isn't some fantastical way of being—it is just being.

EXPERIENCING MINDFUL TRANSFORMATION THROUGH PHENOMENOLOGY

The experience of doing this work was transformational for me. I became a phenomenologist, a writer, and a teacher as a result. I acquired an expanded identity; I see and experience myself differently. I uncovered a self, a being, who was hidden, and acquired new ways of being through learning and practicing phenomenology. While I was learning, exploring, and writing, I discovered an authentic way of being in the world that I had glimmers of, but had been unable to manifest, to fully own.

Being a phenomenologist requires a mindful engagement with phenomena. The phenomena may be the lived experience of self or others, the practice of a profession, the learning of a topic, the experience of art or music, the experience of spirit, the experience of one's physicality, or the experience of the natural world. Being a phenomenologist is a unique way of being-in-the-world that involves releasing our assumptions about the world and engaging directly, mindfully, and fully with whatever is before us. Not only does transformation occur in this process, but it also manifests as mindfulness. While practicing phenomenology, we are, at all times, alert and softly aware of our practice. I changed and I experienced myself changing as I engaged in this work.

Buddhist writers define mindfulness as *choiceless awareness* (Claxton, 1990). Mindfulness is a central concept in Buddhist practice and the desired state to be achieved in many forms of meditation practice. The Buddhist monk Thich Nhat Hanh describes one of the steps of mindfulness:

> The . . . Miracle of Mindfulness is looking deeply. Because you are calm and concentrated [in meditation], you are really there for deep looking. You shine the light of mindfulness on the object of your attention, and at the same time you shine the light of mindfulness on yourself. You observe the object of your attention and you also see your own storehouse full of precious gems. (1975, 66)

In my experience of practicing, mindfulness and phenomenological *looking* are very closely allied. Mindful transformation and phenomenological practice seem to occur in a hermeneutic spiral. Mindful transformation involves living with authentic presence in the natural flow of life. It isn't necessarily about changing oneself to be better in some external sense. It is finding one's own personal truth and living it, simply and clearly. It requires self-knowledge in the psychological and spiritual sense. It requires living purposefully while letting go of absolute knowledge of what this means.

The hermeneutic phenomenological work of experiencing and interpreting the texts of my life created the opportunity for a profound realization of personal transformation. It is the holistic manifold that is often seen when using a hermeneutic spiral of interpretation that creates many layers of experience that lead to the transformation that I discovered.

The transformation I am talking about is a change in consciousness—our awareness of ourselves and ourselves in the world. I believe that every change we approach is ultimately a move toward this new consciousness. We cannot know, before we make a change, what this new way of being will bring into our lives. Knowing this, accepting this, and moving out on the path to transformation anyway was a humbling experience. Learning to be a phenomenologist, practicing mindfulness, taking this learning and practice and trying to be this way while studying and writing about it, and then coming to conclusions from the work were, at times, overwhelming. Sometimes, I was paralyzed for extended periods. Yet, from somewhere deep in my own consciousness, the mindfulness itself allowed me to move into the next spiral of work and understanding.

I end the telling of this story with a sense of humility, and also with a sense of gratitude for my learning and my transformation as I sought to see myself as a phenomenological scholar and practitioner.

REFERENCES

Bentz, Valerie Malhotra. (1989) *Becoming Mature: Childhood Ghosts and Spirits in Adult Life.* New York: Walter de Gruyter.

———. (1995) Husserl, Schutz, "Paul" and Me: Reflections on Writing Phenomenology. *Human Studies, 18,* 41–62.

Bentz, Valerie M., and Jeremy J. Shapiro. (1998) *Mindful Inquiry in Social Research.* Thousand Oaks, CA: Sage.

Claxton, Guy. (1990) *The Heart of Buddhism: Practical Wisdom for an Agitated World.* London: HarperCollins.

Heidegger, Martin. (1962) *Being and Time.* (J. Macquarrie and E. Robinson, Trans.). New York: Harper & Row.

Hultgren, Francine H. (1995) The Phenomenology of "Doing" Phenomenology: The Experience of Teaching and Learning Together. *Human Studies, 18,* 371–38.

Husserl, Edmund. (1965) *Phenomenology and the Crisis of Philosophy.* (Q. Lauer, Trans.) New York: Harper & Row.

Ihde, Don. (1986) *Experimental Phenomenology.* Albany: State University of New York Press.

Jaspers, Karl. (1994) *Basic Philosophical Writings* (rev. ed.). (E. Ehrlich, L. H. Ehrlich, and G. B. Pepper, Trans.) Highlands, NJ: Humanities Press International.

Merleau-Ponty, Maurice. (1962/1979) *Phenomenology of Perception.* (C. Smith, Trans.) Suffolk, UK: St. Edmundsbury Press.

Moustakas, Clark E. (1994) *Phenomenological Research Methods.* Thousand Oaks, CA: Sage.

Nhat Hanh, Thich. (1975) *The Miracle of Mindfulness.* Boston: Beacon Press.

Rehorick, David A. (1986) Shaking the Foundations of Lifeworld: A Phenomenological Account of an Earthquake Experience. *Human Studies, 9,* 379–91.

Rehorick, David, and Gail Taylor. (1995) Thoughtful Incoherence: First Encounters with the Phenomenological-Hermeneutical Domain. *Human Studies, 18*(4), 389–414.

Sartre, Jean-Paul (1956) *Being and Nothingness.* (H. E. Barnes, Trans.) New York: Simon & Schuster.

Schutz, Alfred. (1967) *The Phenomenology of the Social World.* (R. M. Zaner and H. T. Engelhardt, Jr., Trans.) Evanston, IL: Northwestern University Press.

Simpson, Sandra K. (2003) *Mindful Transformation: A Phenomenological Study.* Unpublished Ph.D. dissertation. Santa Barbara, CA: The Fielding Institute.

van Manen, Max. (1990) *Researching Lived Experience: Human Science for an Action Sensitive Pedagogy.* Albany: State University of New York Press.

II

LESSONS FROM ILLNESS AND PERSONAL TRAUMA: PATHWAYS TO INDIVIDUAL CHANGE

4

Trial by Fire

The Transformational Journey of an Adult Male Cancer Survivor

Dudley O. Tower

MY LIFE IN CRISIS, MY TURN TO SCHOLARSHIP

I am a cancer survivor, having been diagnosed with testicular cancer in 1988 at the age of thirty-eight. My treatment included several operations and five months of the most debilitating chemotherapy imaginable. Prior to my diagnosis, I was the chief financial officer of a large automotive systems supplier in the Detroit area. I was very unhappy with my job, where I lived, the people I worked with, and my life in general. I felt trapped by the money and power of my position and regularly drank myself to sleep at night. It was near the end of a long year of intense and emotional merger negotiations that I was diagnosed with cancer. My entire life shifted at the exact moment the doctor told me I had the disease. I was no longer strong, self-assured, and immortal. Two days following my diagnosis, I had my first operation to remove the tumor, and two weeks after that, the infested lymph nodes from my chest and abdomen. Following that was five months of chemotherapy—in the hospital for five gut-wrenching days, five times—until I could stand no more. All of this was followed by months of depression, as I returned to a job and life that had been a primary cause for the disease. Then, finally, I began to feel a glimmer of hope. With the return of my strength came new direction and new priorities.

One year after the end of treatment, I quit my job, intensified my psychotherapy, renewed my relationship with my wife, and first learned of the Ph.D. program at the Fielding Graduate University. In the ensuing years, I remained cancer-free and steadily became more autonomous, adaptable, self-aware, and inclusive in my thinking. My relationships improved, and I began to experience greater meaning in my life. I have had my ups and downs since the cancer, but I have continued to grow. Seventeen years after my brush with mortality, I am still motivated to make the most out of each day. I can truly say that what appeared to be the worst thing that could happen to me at the time was actually the best experience of my life.

In the following essay, I display what coming to phenomenological inquiry has done to help me articulate my experience with cancer and brush with death. In so doing, I offer a wider perspective drawn from the accounts of the men who agreed to co-participate in sharing their stories for my dissertation research. Beyond personal transformation for self and others, my inquiry offers directives and a model to view the conception of cancer survivor in a different and new way.

DEBUNKING MYTHS:
CHALLENGING HABITUATED WAYS OF SEEING

I believe that we have a myth in our society that most cancer survivors remain irreparably damaged by the disease. This myth is perpetuated by the fact that we do not distinguish, in our language or other social symbols, between the long-term survivors of cancer and those people who have been newly diagnosed or recently undergone treatment.

The term *survivor* was used originally to describe the parents of victims of childhood cancer, because there were virtually no actual survivors of cancer until recent years. As survival rates grew, this term was then applied to long-term (more than five years) cancer survivors. However, in more recent years, the term *survivor* has been applied to all people with cancer, from the moment of diagnosis until their death, from any cause. While this presents a perspective of hope for the newly diagnosed and those undergoing treatment, it fails to distinguish those currently experiencing the terror and pain of the disease from those who have had a chance to reflect on these experiences and grow from the process. Several studies dispute this myth of the cancer survivor as victim. These studies actually indicate that a majority of long-term survivors report the same levels of or improvements in their quality of life following the disease (Belec, 1992; Bush, Haberman, Donaldson, and Sullivan, 1995; Haberman, Bush, Young, and Sullivan, 1993; Whedon, Stearns, and Mills, 1995). My study indicates that certain survivors will go beyond mere improvements in their quality of life and actually experience a positive transformation in meaning and consciousness that is the direct result of their survival. However, the lived experience of cancer can be so terrifying, and so devastating, that this transformation never comes easily. For these survivors, their ordeal becomes a turning point of almost mythical proportion—a trial by fire—offering the possibilities of new life on the one hand, and death on the other.

There are alternatives to transformational growth following an experience with cancer, but my study only looked at those adult male survivors who had undergone a self-identified transformation process. However, given the severity and permanent physical effects experienced by some of my co-researchers, and the reaction I get from other survivors when I discuss my findings, I believe a majority of long-term survivors identify with this model. There is something about cancer that is different from other life crises. It will nearly always create the positive changes found in my study, provided a person survives the disease.

STUDYING CANCER SURVIVORSHIP WITH HERMENEUTIC PHENOMENOLOGY

From my life's experience, I wondered about and wanted to study two questions: How are certain people transformed as a result of surviving cancer? What is the transformational experience of being a cancer survivor?

I defined *cancer survivor* as someone who had been disease-free for at least five years, and limited my study to fourteen adult male survivors, ages forty to sixty, who had contracted their cancer as an adult (after twenty-one years of age). I chose to study only men because one of my goals was to better understand my own process of transformation. Men have had a significantly higher lifetime risk of contracting cancer than women (and this risk escalates rapidly with age), and a higher mortality rate from the disease. While there have been several all-female studies of cancer survivorship, my study was the first of its kind to use an all-male group of participants. Since the average male's five-year survival rate from cancer has improved by over 30 percent in the past twenty-five years (National Cancer Institute, 1999), it is becoming increasingly important to understand how men experience their survival from this disease.

It is impossible for someone who has never experienced cancer to truly understand its physical and psychological devastation, or its possible transformational effects. There are certain phenomena that can only be understood by those who have shared the experience, and cancer is one of them. For this reason, I chose hermeneutic phenomenology to study my questions concerning the how and what of cancer and personal transformation. I believed, from the outset, that my own experience of cancer and subsequent personal transformation must be integrated into the analysis to create a thorough and accurate understanding of this phenomenon. Phenomenology provided a framework and worldview that allowed me to interweave my own experience throughout the research process. Instead of

setting aside or hiding my own experience, it became clarified and then integrated in a spiral-like manner with the data to create a continuously
deeper understanding. I allowed the data to change my perceptions and interpretation and, in the end, the research changed me as well, allowing me
to finally integrate this traumatic experience into my life.

Phenomenology is the interpretation of the essence or structure of human experience as it is presented in consciousness. Phenomenology allows
us to reflect upon and interpret the meaning of lived experience by identifying the structural elements, or themes, of the experience in question. The
beauty of phenomenology is that it can make us think, feel, and experience
things that traditional science cannot. The purpose of my research was not
to prove who will become transformed as a result of their cancer, but to
present the possibilities for positive change following cancer, and describe
how a person might possibly turn the worst thing that ever happened to
them into the best.

The second part of my methodology, hermeneutics, addresses how we
understand and interpret the meaning of written texts. According to Paul
Ricoeur,

> to understand is to understand oneself in front of the text. It is not a question
> of imposing upon the text our finite capacity of understanding, but of expos-
> ing ourselves to the text and receiving from it an enlarged self. (1981, 143)

The concept of the *hermeneutic spiral* was critical to my methodology, and
involved a process of moving back and forth between my own experience
and prior interpretation of the phenomenon, the relevant literature on the
subject, and co-researcher interview data (see Bentz and Shapiro, 1998,
chapters 3 and 8). This inevitably resulted in a new interpretation, which
became the basis for a next spiral, and so on. I intentionally stretched my
interpretations of the data through the use of intuition in search of the underlying structural themes, and ultimately this process resulted in a written
text describing the phenomenon. The written text also changed and clarity
was enhanced through a process of writing and rewriting.

TRAUMA AND TRANSFORMATION

The term *personal transformation* is most often associated with positive
growth or development, defined by Rogers as the "formative directional
tendency . . . toward greater order, greater complexity, greater interrelated-
ness" (1980, 133). For our purposes, it is useful to think of transformational change as occurring relatively rapidly, as opposed to so-called normal
adult development, which most often evolves slowly over the course of a

person's lifetime. Taking all of these factors together, we can view personal transformation as involving significant and rapid changes of a positive developmental nature.

While most theories of human development assume a slow, continuous growth toward higher stages of complexity (for example, Erikson, 1980, 1982; Kegan, 1982, 1994; Labouvie-Vief, 1982), it is possible that many people develop in the fits and starts that more closely follow the ups and downs of circumstances in their lives (Tower, 2000). The types of life experience that might catalyze periods of rapid growth could involve positive new opportunities, circumstances, or challenges, but growth might also be triggered by extreme stress, traumatic events, or life crises. There is a great deal of support, in the literature of posttraumatic growth, for the idea that transformational growth is often catalyzed by extreme trauma; the literature also reveals some insights into how these changes come about.

According to the newly emerging theory of posttraumatic growth, and other cognitive learning theories, meaning, awareness, our interpretation of experience, our sense of safety, and self-concept are all created by previously formed structures of expectation, alternatively called *meaning perspectives* (Mezirow, 1991), *frames of reference* (McCann and Pearlman, 1990), *basic assumptions* (Janoff-Bulman, 1992), and *schemas*. The deepest of these mental structures are heavily defended and resistant to change. However, due to the life-threatening nature of certain traumatic events, such as cancer, our defenses can be bypassed and these mental structures ruptured, forcing the reconstruction of a new set of mental structures.

Rapid personal growth, or transformation, occurs in the positive reconstruction of these mental structures (Tedeschi and Calhoun, 1995). Certain aspects of positive growth, resulting from a more realistic understanding of one's own mortality (limitations, priorities, and purpose), will nearly always follow trauma or life crisis. However, this realization might also be accompanied by feelings of fear and anxiety (Janoff-Bulman, 1992; Lifton, 1979), denial, and other forms of resistance (Yalom, 1980). The degree of change experienced will depend on several factors, including previous trauma history, posttrauma environment, timing of any therapeutic intervention, as well as the person's self-capacities and ego resources (McCann and Pearlman, 1990). Other factors impacting the change process are the extent to which survivors respond to their trauma as a major challenge (O'Leary, 1998) and remain engaged in the change process (Carver, 1998), an ability to tolerate distressing emotions, an ability to integrate the experience into one's existing mental structures creatively, and the support of others (Janoff-Bulman, 1992). In addition, the experience of extreme growth or personal transformation will depend on the initial pretrauma physical and psychosocial starting conditions of the person.

PHENOMENOLOGICAL THEMES:
INSIGHTS FROM THE MEN'S ACCOUNTS

My research clearly supports a model of survivor transformation having five distinct stages and thirteen themes, beginning with a downward spiral of increasing disaffection and despair prior to the diagnosis, and ending with a life full of new hope, relationships, and possibilities. The five stages are *initial conditions, diagnosis, treatment, transition,* and *integration.* It is important to understand the transformation process of long-term cancer survivors in terms of the totality of this five-stage model. This is because there is one very dreadful reality for the survivor if we look only at the beginning of this process, while there is another, most often positive, reality for those who live through the entire process taken as a whole. With this in mind, I present the model and selected themes from the data collected (Tower, 2000). I refer to my study participants as *co-researchers* since my individual experience links me to their lifeworlds in a way that renders us equals, not researcher versus participants.

Our biggest misconception about cancer is that we tend to view it as an event, unconnected to a past or a future. However, for many male survivors, their cancer is experienced as a turning point in a journey, a trial by fire, as noted above. This journey often begins long before the onset of cancer, and, in my experience, with a steady slide into despair and hopelessness. Under these conditions, cancer can represent a bottoming out of this downward spiral that, if overcome, creates within a survivor the power to change his life. Two co-researchers expressed it this way:

> I don't look at my cancer experience now as if it were an event. Instead I view it as a journey. It is one of those milestones that hits you in your life, like when you discover your calling, or something that just makes you face the basic truths. . . . I looked at it as an adventure, something to be learned from.

> I have, and continue to view this experience as a journey, one that will end only when I die. It feels like the type of changes I have made are in line with some universal sense of human purpose; that this is what we were meant to be doing with our lives, not simply procreating, working at meaningless jobs, and making money.

In this manner, cancer can become the course correction in a life story that shifts our consciousness, moving one from meaninglessness to a life full of meaning, and from the direction of others to increasing self-direction. With this understanding of the model as a journey, each stage dependent upon the other, rather than a series of events, I next discuss each of the model's five stages and selections from the underlying themes.

Stage 1: Initial Conditions

The literature on posttraumatic growth indicates that good initial mental health will positively affect a person's response to trauma, while poor initial mental health, or neuroticism, will be a detriment to positive growth (Tennen and Affleck, 1998, 72–73). The results of my study dispute this contention. My co-researchers who reported lower levels of personal transformation following their cancer were also those who reported the most connection and best adjustment prior to contracting the disease. Conversely, I found those co-researchers who reported discontent, increasing alienation, and even varying levels of neuroticism in their precancer lives were also those who reported greater levels of positive transformation following their cancer.

One theme within stage 1 is *alienation* (for linkage to cancer depression and Type-A personality, see Carver and Humphries, 1982; Friedman and Booth-Kewley, 1987). In nearly all cases, the precancer lives of my co-researchers were stressful, taken for granted, unsatisfying, out of touch with their real needs, overly identified with traditional cultural conceptions of masculinity, and fearful. For many of these men, their cancer represented the bottoming out in a long process of increasing withdrawal and isolation from the outside world, and served as a turning point in their lives. Viewed from this perspective, increasing alienation and despair might be viewed as an opportunity for transformation of meaning and consciousness by forcing a crisis.

Stage 2: Diagnosis

The diagnosis of cancer nearly always comes as a complete surprise, shattering our self-concept and destroying our every vision of the future. There is very little in the literature on the actual moment of trauma, the shattering of an assumptive world (Janoff-Bulman, 1992), that can also lead to a transformation in consciousness.

Existential terror was a theme that characterized the stage of diagnosis. In each and every case, my co-researchers described their diagnosis as a complete surprise, in spite of many early warning signs. Yet each co-researcher also instantly recognized that the diagnosis was correct, as if, at some level, they knew it all along. In all these cases, including my own, I am convinced that it was this single moment of diagnostic terror that shattered the mind's assumptive barriers, laying the groundwork for a positive transformational change in mental structures. Three men expressed it this way:

> I was dead. When I first heard the diagnosis, I didn't know what to do. I was completely devastated. It was the farthest thing from my mind.

Terror, Terror. It was the "C" word. I remember I was obsessed with it. My re-action to first being diagnosed with cancer was like stepping into an elevator shaft without the elevator being there. "I have what? I'm going to die."

And that just about knocked me off the chair. "Cancer," and right away, it's like "Oh, my God, what does this mean, I'm dying." What does this mean to me, my marriage, my life?

The moment of diagnosis is so terrifying, and therefore so significant in the survivor's journey, that it deserves its own stage in this process. However, for most survivors, their ordeal is only beginning.

Stage 3: Treatment

Although the moment of diagnosis is usually the most terrifying stage in a survivor's journey, the actual physical trauma usually takes place in the treatment of the disease. During this stage, the survivor is faced with the prospect of future surgeries, chemotherapy, radiation, and hormone treat-ment. He is entering the treatment tunnel and cannot see any light at its end. However, as if his treatment options were not enough, he is also faced with other important matters, such as where to go for treatment, how to pay for it, career implications, insurance considerations, lost wages, disability, wills, the family's future, guilt, and so much more. To understand the depths from which a survivor must eventually emerge in order to transform himself, one must understand this period of treatment, because it can ex-tend a survivor's physical and mental suffering over an almost intolerable period of time, completely destroying any remaining potential the mind has to maintain its prior identity and illusions.

Fives themes characterize the treatment stage: *horrors of medicine, time for reflection, letting go of control, redefining positive attitude,* and *a time for love.* The *horrors of medicine* theme includes the *acute stage,* which begins at diag-nosis and continues through the initial courses of surgery, chemotherapy, and radiation treatments. Here is how some individuals expressed it:

Chemotherapy brings a person about as close to death as you can be without actually dying. You feel like you are dying. You look like you are dying. And sometimes you wish you were dead.

It was undoubtedly the worst experience of my whole life. It got to the point where I couldn't move, I couldn't get out of bed, I couldn't even talk some-times. Sometimes I would have to write out a note if I wanted something.

Then, there are the problems of *long-term* and *late* effects, which the survivor must continue to deal with, sometimes for a lifetime (Hoffman, 1996).

Most important to the transformation that will come has been the dissolution of any sense of self he might have had prior to the cancer.

A time for reflection is often an important opening in a survivor's life. A key to the transformation of a cancer survivor's meaning structures is having the time and ability to reflect critically on any distorted assumptions, and how they might have constrained or been indirectly responsible for his illness (Mezirow, 1991). This reflection process is facilitated by the trauma experienced during this stage, because the survivor's defenses are down; there is simply nothing left to defend. As one survivor said,

> now, all of a sudden, I couldn't do anything. So I had a lot of time on my hands and I started doing some reading, some praying, some meditating. During that time, during the reflection, I began to view myself differently, and view my experience differently.

What is so devastating about cancer, especially in this stage, also provides the survivor with an opportunity for growth. Cancer forces the survivor to *let go of control,* the third theme of the treatment stage. There is only so much the survivor can actually control, and, over everything else, he must learn to let go. This frees the survivor from unnecessary fear and worry, letting go of future plans that are not congruent with current conditions. This allows him to connect with new people, new experiences, and new capabilities. This reversal of the controlling behavior, that so dominated many lives prior to the cancer, was another key building block in the transformational process experienced by each of these survivors.

At the time of my study, I was concerned about even discussing the concept of positive attitude with other cancer survivors. *Redefining positive attitude* is the next theme of the stage of treatment. I had friends who died from cancer, suffering all the while with a smile on their faces, intent on showing the world what a positive attitude they had. I viewed this type of positive attitude as a front, a façade, depleting my friends' energies and creating stress rather than helping them to fight the disease. However, in spite of my preconceptions, one of my co-researchers embodied a positive attitude as he defeated small-cell lung cancer over thirty years ago, against all odds. His comments provide us with an idea of the lived experience of positive attitude:

> No, I wasn't concerned. And to be honest about it, I was never concerned for my life the whole time I had the cancer. I didn't think about dying at all. I never had that idea in my mind that I wasn't going to make it. I knew I was going to make it. Why? I don't know.

Positive attitude, then, for the purposes of surviving cancer, is not a quality easily learned. A survivor cannot simply adopt this attitude for himself, and he should not try to adopt this attitude in order to please others. This type of positive attitude is characterized by optimism and hope. It means not accepting the social construction that cancer equals death. It involves an ability always to see the possibilities in a situation, to view illness as an opportunity for growth, and to remain engaged throughout the healing process.

A time for love is the final treatment stage. The single most important variable impacting a survivor's transformational process is social support (Beardslee, 1989; Calhoun and Tedeschi, 1998; Fawcett, 1994; Hirshberg and Barasch, 1995; Janoff-Bulman, 1992). I had always interpreted this need for support as a one-way street. I was surprised to interview so many men who experienced their cancer as an opportunity to move closer to their spouses and children. Personal transformation following cancer is related not only to the support a survivor receives during his illness and recovery, but also his ability to reciprocate the love and support he receives from others.

Stage 4: Transition

In my own experience, there was a period following treatment during which I was depressed, wanted to withdraw from social contact with other people, had little interest in work or other activities, had thoughts of moving to a remote location, was in denial of the ongoing threat to my life, and avoided stressful encounters of all kinds. No one ever told me to expect this period of early transition, and certainly no one told me it was all right (or even normal) to have these feelings. Instead, I thought there was something terribly and permanently wrong with me.

My research revealed that *depression and withdrawal* is a major theme of the transition stage. The survivor has just left one stage in his journey where his entire being has been focused on getting through a horrible treatment and staying alive. The expectation is for things to get much better, provided one can only get through the treatment stage. However, the survivor's reality is something quite different. Instead of things immediately getting better, he finds that friends and family are treating him differently, the medical support has gone on to another active case, and there is a problem adjusting to the effects of the disease and its treatment. He must now resume a normal life, in spite of having to deal with the stigma of the disease, concerns regarding insurance and employability, fear of the cancer returning, anger, and strange emotional problems such as depression, inferiority, and guilt. The survivor feels extreme pressure at this stage, from himself as well as friends and family, to get on with his life, to put the cancer behind him. Two men shared their sense of what re-entry felt like:

> I tried to go back to work. I did go back to work as quickly as my physical body would heal, but I found that I couldn't concentrate. I felt weak. I felt more than

weak: defeated, black. I didn't know where to turn, how to get on the other side of this.

As I look back, I became horrifically depressed. It's not just the medical part, the physical rupture. It's the real pressure to "get on with your life," "you must be grateful," and all that.

The posttreatment cancer survivor is at his lowest point in the journey. It is a time of maximum ego disruption, and the survivor frequently has little or no remaining self-esteem. The survivor is full of shame; in his mind, he is now only a shell of his former self. Emotional, without goals, and hiding from all external influences, the survivor is extremely vulnerable, and many men are lured back into their prior worlds, which can now seem like a living death. However, others learn to dwell for a time in this state of nothingness, holding, for as long as they can, a dynamic tension between transformation and psychological pain, to emerge positively changed.

Positive stress is a second theme of the transition stage. Koocher and O'Malley (1981) coined the metaphor *Damocles syndrome* to describe the continuing, long-term stress experienced by survivors of childhood cancer. The picture of a giant sword hanging over the heads of cancer survivors for the rest of their lives is, in many cases, accurate. However, I dispute the contention of most cancer researchers that all stress has a negative effect on the survivor and, instead, believe that, in many cases, stress can have a positive impact on personal growth. In my opinion, the most compelling explanation as to how posttreatment stress levels can serve as a catalyst for personal growth comes from Lifton's (1979) discussion of the survivor's *death imprint*. Most of my co-researchers were intensely aware of their vulnerability to future cancer, and were using that awareness to make positive changes and live more meaningful lives.

The doctor put me on a three-month follow-up schedule for the next three years and then on a six-month for the next two years. Now I see him at six months, and then the next six months I see the internist. It will go this way for the rest of my life, because my form of cancer can go into remission for long periods.

This fear can be repressed, or it can be acknowledged and used to motivate positive change.

Stage 5: Integration

The transitional stage in a survivor's journey can last a few months or many years. There is some evidence that the longer a person can remain in this transitional stage, the greater will be his personal growth. Eventually, however, the survivor will reconstruct the mental structures that have been shattered by the disease, consolidate his cancer experience into a congruent life history, and achieve a new equilibrium that integrates the survivor's gains and losses into a higher-order level of consciousness. This is, most frequently, the final stage in the survivor's journey: a time when the majority of pain and trauma are behind the survivor, the limitations caused by the disease have either been corrected or adjusted to, the memories of the ordeal are fading into the past, and the survivor is ready to consolidate his gains from the experience and proceed confidently on with his life. A majority of those who live to become long-term survivors of this disease will be positively transformed by it.

Transformative growth is the next theme of the integration stage. In my own experience of being diagnosed with cancer, certain changes were immediate and automatic. Before my diagnosis, I felt trapped in a joyless and stressful job, in a world where career was the most important thing. Immediately, my job and career became unimportant, the love I had for my wife and my own personal health became the focus of my concentration, and all the little things that used to annoy me about my own life, other people, and circumstances were no longer of major consequence. I can't describe it any other way than to say that I suddenly got *the big picture*. It was like opening a door and moving instantly from a little world into a much larger one. This realization was sudden, automatic, and lasting. This immediate existential realization is similar to what White referred to as a *course correction* in people who have near-death experiences (1997).

I clearly view the transformational growth of cancer survivors differently than a majority of authors and researchers on this subject. Most descriptions of transformation following trauma are static conceptualizations of distinct types of change (such as improved relationships) that do not adequately represent the continuing development of those sudden, initial changes experienced by the survivor, as they evolve over the course of his entire journey. I tend to view the transformation process of a cancer survivor as a dynamic process, beginning at the moment of that initial course correction in the diagnosis/early treatment stages, and extending indefinitely into the survivor's future. This excerpt from my personal accounts captures the idea:

> I look at it as sort of an awakening. I feel more alive since my cancer than before. More aware of what's going on inside of me and around me; more alive to the present moment.

The changes experienced by many male survivors begin with an existential realization that one's life has been largely a socially scripted act up to that point. The sudden clarity of this understanding results in an automatic shift

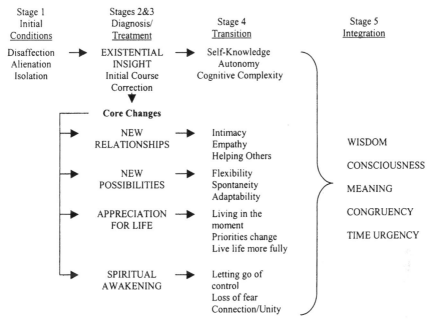

Figure 4.1. The Transformational Journey of an Adult Male Cancer Survivor

in priorities leading to improved relationships, becoming more appreciative of life, seeing new possibilities for one's actions, and possibly a new emphasis on spirituality. These initial changes do not remain static as the literature suggests. These changes continue to develop into the integration stage of the model, wherein the survivor has the potential to find his authentic self and discover new meaning and purpose to his life, a sense of congruency, an expanded sense of connection with other people and the world around him, and the consciousness of a strong, realistic, and nondefensive sense of self.

The change and transformation during the course of a cancer survivor's journey are summarized and depicted in Figure 4.1.

RE-ENVISIONING CANCER: SOME CONTRIBUTIONS FROM PHENOMENOLOGICAL INQUIRY

There is a misconception about how most of us view cancer. It is certainly a catastrophe for many but, for those of us who survive the experience, it can lead to a transformation in meaning and consciousness. This study was the first of its kind to look exclusively at the positive psychosocial transformation of long-term, adult-male cancer survivors. The hermeneutic-phenomenological methodology that I employed during the research allowed me to integrate into the study my own experience of surviving and then being transformed by cancer. This led to a greater understanding of the phenomenon than I could have ever achieved using more conventional scientific research methods. Additionally, my co-researchers responded differently to me than if I were some dispassionate researcher. They confided in me. They trusted me. They knew I could understand and empathize.

The results of this research include a model of survivor transformation, describing the journey of a cancer survivor beginning prior to his disease, extending through diagnosis and treatment, a long transition period, and finally into a stage of integration and transformation. Several of my more specific findings, discovered in the analysis of themes, run counter to the prevailing wisdom and practice regarding cancer survivorship, and I hope they will inform other survivors and the healthcare community. I hope my findings will provide a basis for new action by this community, facilitating the survivor's recovery and personal growth following treatment.

New symbols of survivorship are necessary if we are to accurately distinguish the growing group of long-term survivors from the victims of this disease. The essence of my research, and of my own experience of cancer survivorship, is captured in this holistic view of a life transformed, as expressed by one of my fellow searchers and co-researchers:

> If it wasn't for the cancer, I never would have realized how wonderful and precious life is. I don't think that most people ever really get a feel for how precious life is until they have an experience where they almost die. I don't think I would be nearly as appreciative of the things that I have, the place I live, the place I work, and the country I live in without that experience. And I appreciate the beauty of nature now and realize it is something special. I don't treat it like it's going to be there forever and can therefore wait and enjoy it later. The biggest thing I don't do anymore is take life for granted.

REFERENCES

Beardslee, William R. (1989) The Role of Self-Understanding in Resilient Individuals: The Development of a Perspective. *American Journal of Orthopsychiatry, 59*(2), 266–78.

Belec, Ruth H. (1992) Quality of Life: Perceptions of Long-Term Survivors of Bone Marrow Transplantation. *Oncology Nursing Forum, 19*(1), 31–37.

Bentz, Valerie Malhotra, and Jeremy J. Shapiro. (1998) *Mindful Inquiry in Social Research*. Thousand Oaks, CA: Sage.

Bush, N. E., Mel Haberman, Gary Donaldson, and Keith M. Sullivan. (1995) Quality of Life of 125 Adults Surviving 6–18 Years after Bone Marrow Transplantation. *Social Science and Medicine, 40*(4), 479–90.

Calhoun, Lawrence G., and Richard G. Tedeschi. (1998) Beyond Recovery from Trauma: Implications for Clinical Practice and Research. *Journal of Social Issues, 54*(2), 357–71.

Carver, Charles S. (1998) Resilience and Thriving: Issues, Models, and Linkages. *Journal of Social Issues, 54*(2), 245–66.

Carver, Charles S., and Charlene Humphries. (1982) Social Psychology of the Type A coronary-Prone Behavior Pattern. In G. S. Sanders and J. Suls (Eds.), *Social Psychology of Health and Illness* (33–64). Hillsdale, NJ: Lawrence Erlbaum.

Erikson, Erik H. (1980) *Identity and the Life Cycle.* New York: W.W. Norton.

———. (1982) *The Life Cycle Completed: A Review.* New York: W.W. Norton.

Fawcett, J. (1994) *A Computer-Based Survey of Cancer Survivors.* Oncolink (University of Pennsylvania Cancer Center). Retrieved June 1, 1999, from http://www.oncolink.org/psychosocial/survivor.html.

Friedman, Howard S., and Stephanie Booth-Kewley. (1987) The "Disease-Prone Personality:" A Meta-Analytic View of the Construct. *American Psychologist, 42*(6), 539–55.

Haberman, Mel, N. Bush, K. Young, and Keith M. Sullivan. (1993) Quality of Life of Adult Long-Term Survivors of Bone Marrow Transplantation: A Qualitative Analysis of Narrative Data. *Oncology Nursing Forum, 20*(10), 1545–53.

Hirshberg, Caryle, and Marc I. Barasch. (1995) *Remarkable Recovery: What Extraordinary Healings Tell Us about Getting Well and Staying Well.* New York: Riverhead Books.

Hoffman, B. (Ed.). (1996) *A Cancer Survivor's Almanac: Charting Your Journey.* Minneapolis, MN: Chronimed.

Janoff-Bulman, Ronnie. (1992) *Shattered Assumptions: Towards a New Psychology of Trauma.* New York: The Free Press.

Kegan, Robert. (1982) *The Evolving Self: Problem and Process in Human Development.* Cambridge, MA: Harvard University Press.

———. (1994) *In Over Our Heads: The Mental Demands of Modern Life.* Cambridge, MA: Harvard University Press.

Koocher, Gerald P., and John E. O'Malley. (1981) *The Damocles Syndrome: Psychosocial Consequences of Surviving Childhood Cancer.* New York: McGraw-Hill.

Labouvie-Vief, Gisela. (1982) Dynamic Development and Mature Autonomy: A Theoretical Prologue. *Human Development,* 25, 161–91.

Lifton, Robert J. (1979) *The Broken Connection: On Death and the Continuity of Life.* Washington, DC: American Psychiatric Press.

McCann, I. Lisa, and Laurie A. Pearlman. (1990) *Psychological Trauma and the Adult Survivor: Theory, Therapy, and Transformation.* New York: Brunner/Mazel.

Mezirow, Jack. (1991) *Transformative Dimensions of Adult Learning.* San Francisco: Jossey-Bass.

National Cancer Institute. (1999) *SEER Cancer Statistics Review, 1973–1996 "Initial Content" Section 1—Overview* (Online). Retrieved December 1, 1999, from http://www-seer.ims.nci.nih.gov/Publications/CSR1973_1996/overview/overview19b.pdf.

O'Leary, Virginia E. (1998) Strength in the Face of Adversity: Individual and Social Thriving. *Journal of Social Issues, 54*(2), 425–46.

Ricoeur, Paul. (1981) *Hermeneutics and the Human Sciences.* (J. B. Thompson, Ed. and Trans.) Cambridge: Cambridge University Press.

Rogers, Carl R. (1980) *A Way of Being.* Boston: Houghton Mifflin.

Tedeschi, Richard G., and Lawrence G. Calhoun. (1995). *Trauma and Transformation: Growing in the Aftermath of Suffering.* Thousand Oaks, CA: Sage.

Tennen, Howard, and Glenn Affleck. (1998) Personality and Transformation in the Face of Adversity. In R. G. Tedeschi, C. L. Park, and L. G. Calhoun (Eds.), *Posttraumatic Growth: Positive Changes in the Aftermath of Crisis* (65–98). Mahwah, NJ: Lawrence Erlbaum.

Tower, Dudley. (2000) *Trans-Survivorship: The Cancer Survivor's Journey from Trauma to Transformation.* Unpublished Ph.D. Dissertation. Santa Barbara, CA: Fielding Graduate Institute.

Whedon, M., D. Stearns, and L. E. Mills. (1995) Quality of Life of Long-Term Adult Survivors of Autologous Bone Marrow Transplantation. *Oncology Nursing Forum,* 22(10), 1527–35.

White, Patti R. (1997) The Anatomy of a Transformation: An Analysis of the Psychological Structure of Four Near-Death Experiences. *Journal of Near-Death Studies, 15* (3), 163–85.

Yalom, Irving D. (1980) *Existential Psychotherapy.* New York: Basic Books.

5

My Body the Traitor

Fearing a Recurrence of Breast Cancer

Roanne Thomas-MacLean

Diane (a pseudonym): I think there is going to come a time, when the tamoxifen is over . . . that I am going to think, "Oh God, what do I do?" I don't know how you deal with it. I guess you just, each day, kind of take it and keep it in perspective and figure, if you got through five years, well, then you can get through another five. But I think it is going to be a problem, because there will be, "What am I doing now? Is it [cancer] really gone?" And there is no way to know. You do your examination every month, and generally feel good, but you know your body has betrayed you once and it could do it again.

What does it mean to experience the constancy of fear associated with the possibility of breast cancer recurrence? What provokes this fear? What is the meaning of fear within the context of surviving breast cancer? Exploring the phenomenon of fear illustrates the interconnection of body, mind, and society, as fear may engender a physical response that is not easily separated from cognitive experience, or from one's social environment. Fear may involve sweaty palms, a racing heartbeat, nausea, trembling, and muscle tension, as well as a racing of thoughts that unexpectedly surface in rapid-fire succession. Further, fear may be experienced as a response to a particular social event, such as public speaking or flying. Fear can be experienced as a fleeting or brief moment of panic that ends when a situation is resolved, but some experiences of fear may be more constant, or may be described as simmering.

As a researcher and a teacher, phenomenology has provided me with an opportunity to explore complex topics such as fear. In this chapter, I describe how embodiment may be conceptualized phenomenologically, and offer illustrative excerpts from my study of fear in women who are recovering from breast cancer (Thomas, 1994). I explore how women experience both body and culture as traitorous, following diagnoses of breast cancer, along with the ways in which participants describe their bodies as suspect. I close with a commentary on the transformational nature of phenomenological inquiry for me, for healthcare practitioners, and, I hope, for increasing numbers of physicians.

PUTTING EMBODIMENT AT THE CENTER

Susan: I do keep a closer watch on the other breast now and I'm very, you know, I can get very paranoid. If there's a tiny lump, I'm right there to the doctor.

Roanne: Do you ever think about the possibility of a recurrence?

Janice: All the time. And I think if any cancer patient told you they didn't, they'd be lying.

It may be argued that all of our knowledge is held bodily because it is through our bodies that we are rooted in the world (Bentz and Shapiro, 1998). Central to Merleau-Ponty's phenomenology are the concepts of embodiment and lived experience, ideas first introduced by Husserl. Embodiment is understood as an aspect of being, and people do not simply have bodies, but they are their bodies (Rehorick, 1986). Understanding embodiment means understanding "persons as they are in their world within their body, which is consciously finding expression in feeling, speech, thought, sensing, judging, and so on" (Parker as cited in Munhall, 1994, 291).

Despite scholars' increasing interests in body and embodiment, certain aspects of embodiment still have not been explored. Bordo writes "we are more in touch with our bodies than ever before. But at the same time, they have become alienated products, texts of our own creative making" (1993, 288). Further, Gatens writes that "recent feminist research suggests that the history of Western thought shows a deep hatred and fear of the body" (1996, 68). As a result, within the discipline of sociology, *body* has been neglected as an area of inquiry. Within the realm of phenomenology, however, body is viewed as integral to self, a view that has been shared by the people I have interviewed in the context of my own research.

Leder writes that phenomenology allows researchers to suspend scientific, or positivistic, ideas about body,

> to allow for an encounter with the phenomena of our daily experience . . . experientially, our body is very *different* than other physical objects in the world. . . . When the body falls sick, we are left not simply with a broken machine, but with a world transformed. (1992a, 5)

Leder continues: "through hearing the patient's *story*, one comes to know in detail of her world as she embodies it. . . . Only in this broader context will the full significance and etiology of her illness emerge" (1992b, 29).

EMBODIED EXPERIENCES OF BREAST CANCER: PHENOMENOLOGICAL ACCOUNTS OF FEAR

The neglect of embodiment and the cultural context of breast cancer imply that women have had little opportunity to express their experiences of fear of recurrence after breast cancer. Mathieson asserts that biomedical language does not sufficiently address women's experiences of illness and that "women speaking for themselves about their illness have suggested a far richer level of description" (1994, 52).

I turned to women with firsthand knowledge of the meaning of breast cancer to illustrate the significance of this illness and its impact on embodiment (Thomas, 1994). I interviewed twelve breast cancer survivors on two occasions each, for a total of twenty-four interviews. The number of years that had passed since diagnosis ranged from one to twenty-four. Breast cancer treatments included mastectomy, radiation, and chemotherapy, as well as combinations of these three modalities. Although a number of themes emerged from my analysis, I will elaborate here only on the theme of fear as captured by each of my participants.

Through their stories, participants show how illness transforms embodiment through the experience of fear. Susan said, following her biopsy, that there was cancer at the edge of the site, so she chose to have a mastectomy, mostly because she did not want to have to worry about or monitor her body for a recurrence. However, Susan went on to describe a process for monitoring her body. When asked if she worries about recurrence, Susan replied that it is only when she has nothing to do and it is quiet that it occurs to her.

Beth talked of the way she is followed closely by her doctor, so that "it doesn't develop into anything that gets away from us." She had been talking about the possibility that there was still breast tissue remaining at the site of her mastectomy, so "it" could be referring to her body or also the unknown of cancer. Diane's words introduced the theme of betrayal as she talked about monitoring her body:

> *Diane*: I guess that I would say that, before I had breast cancer, I never really thought about my body that much; now, I guess I know it's something that can betray you, without you even knowing what's going on. Because there were no symptoms, there was no feeling ill, or pain, or any problem; then, all of a sudden, there's something just there. I think it makes you a little more stressed out.

What's it going to do next? Not only what's it going to do next, but there's probably nothing I can do to stop it if it decides it's going to spread. I think it makes you a little more, "Are you going to get something else?" It also makes you, before, if I had an ache or a pain somewhere, I'd say, "Oh, I just pulled something." Now, when you have it, you think all sorts of other thoughts, so if there's pain somewhere you think, "What's happening here?" or "Why is this doing that?" It's sort of like when I was on a business trip, when my hand swelled, if I'd never had breast cancer, I'd just think, "It's hot," or "I pulled something," and it's fine. But you start to think other things; so, I think, probably I'd say that I don't trust my body as much as I used to.

Susan, Beth, and Diane felt that both health and illness can be understood as processes that do not end with the completion of treatment (see Watson, 1988).

Compounding the fear of recurrence is the fear of being too fearful of it. Women express the idea that they do not wish to be controlled by their anxiety about recurrence. Diane showed how a fear of recurrence, or not wishing to be controlled by fear, is linked to habitual embodiment. Diane stated that she was prepared to make some changes to her diet and lifestyle as a result of breast cancer, but that she was also not prepared to change other aspects of her life:

Diane: I'm prepared to make some accommodation and I do. . . . I try to eat healthier. . . . I did lose the weight that I gained, and I do try to eat healthier and make sure I don't get overtired, which is always easy to say, but not easy to do. I changed my work habits a little. What I won't change is certain other lifestyle issues people talk about. We like to entertain, so we do that fairly frequently, and entertaining doesn't have to involve alcohol, but I like to have a drink. . . . Some of the research says probably you shouldn't be consuming alcohol. So far I haven't made that choice. . . . I guess you are responsible for your own body to some extent, but I guess when I said I'm not prepared to make those lifestyle changes, I work hard; if that's what I like for enjoyment, that's what I'll do.

The cultural roots of fear are inextricably connected to embodiment. Janice demonstrated the ways in which a fear of recurrence are linked to cultural context. She demonstrated an awareness of healthcare cutbacks and the limitations of medicine when she talked about her decision to have a second mastectomy:

Janice: The way our medical system is today, you might have to wait a month before you get in there to have it removed, so you could be almost dead in a month. It could spread into the lymph system and all through your body in a month.

Past, present, and future are all experienced in the immediacy of fear. Fear of recurrence connects the past, present, and future in body's immediacy. Of time, Merleau-Ponty notes, "what is past or future for me is present in the world" (1962, 412).

Arlene said that the fear of recurrence "is with you twenty-four hours a day. It never leaves." Marie described similar feelings:

Marie: I don't know; maybe I'm a lot more inquisitive now, trying to see what the future holds for me. I don't worry about it, but I am very aware; let's say that it has happened and can happen. So, therefore, enjoy every day that you have that you feel well. And basically, I do feel well. But like, you'd go to the oncologist, and . . . that's something I'd never experienced. To go visit the on- cologist, you have to go to the oncology clinic. While you're sitting there, wait- ing for your appointment, there's people there with no hair, and there's people there very frail, and it's, you know, you're aware that could happen. That could happen to anybody; but I'd never considered it could happen to me before, so that's a little different.

Medical professionals have the ability or potential to alleviate feelings of vulnerability, fear, and marginalization. Seeing the oncologist and learning that she is well makes Marie feel very secure. For Arlene, regular tests pro- vide her with a sense of relief when she learns the results. Fran stated that she now wishes she had had a radical rather than a modified radical mas- tectomy, because it would alleviate some of her fears of recurrence. She says, of her fear,

Fran: I think about it . . . think about it coming back, whether I'll have breast cancer, bone cancer, or what. Not necessarily that I'll get it again, but you never know.

Illness is associated with disempowerment. Is this what is feared? What further damage to body and self could illness inflict if it were to return? Van Manen states that, when body calls us to attention through illness or "something conspicuous," such as an unfamiliar ache or pain, "we exist in a protracted state of 'dis-ease,' literally uneasiness" (1998, ¶42). Together with my participants, I recognize what Leder (1990) describes as the elu- siveness of the body and our lack of knowledge about physiological di- mensions of the body. Past experiences of body, as well as body's inherent mysteries, fuel fear.

Janice illustrated these ideas when she talked about her decision to have a mastectomy rather than a lumpectomy; Beth expressed a similar sentiment.

Janice: If there's still breast tissue there, it's a chance for cancer . . . remove it, because I couldn't live with it there and I can sure live without it. . . . So, maybe it was a coward's way out . . . but it really wasn't a hard decision to make be- cause, I just figured, get rid of them and then I wouldn't have to worry.

Beth: So, leaving the breast there, this could occur again, and we wouldn't know, and maybe it would have advanced a lot further before we did realize, so it was best to take it then.

Of body, Toombs writes that, simultaneously, "I am responsible for it, yet at its disposal, and at the same time it expresses and embodies me. My body is at once the most intimate yet alien presence" (1992, 61). Body is both powerful and powerless. Like the women who participated in my study, I can make decisions about my body, but I am also acutely aware that I am at my body's mercy.

Once a woman has had breast cancer, what Olesen terms *trivia* takes on more significance. Olesen describes *mundane ailments* as those that are ordinary or everyday occurrences, such as an "ache, pain, discomfort [or] rash" (1992, 210). Even without experience of a serious illness, Olesen states, such ailments can induce feelings of vulnerability. Yet vulnerability has not been a focus of research. What does it mean to be vulnerable? To be vulnerable may be defined as "able to be hurt or wounded or injured" as well as "unprotected, exposed to danger" (Hawkins, 1987, 759). These meanings imply that being vulnerable represents a possibility of being victimized. Is a fear of recurrence illustrative of women's experiences of victimization as a result of breast cancer? How might we understand victimization separate from some of its social constructs, which imply that victims are to blame for their circumstances? Victimization is a form of suffering. Synonymous with suffering are experiences such as grieving and sorrow. Breast cancer represents a loss of what has been taken for granted—a loss not only of health, but of connections with others that have been irrevocably altered, along with the connections to body:

Janice: It [breast cancer] is always there in the back of your mind, like, I have to go twice a year, once in Saint John and once to the surgeon, and the night before I go to Saint John, I'm always nerved up, that whole week before. I'm always nerved up because you always think, "Okay, are they going to find something?" They never do. I guess you just have to have faith. But it does get hard, because it's always there, in the back of your mind, always. You might not even realize it's there, but find a lump and it's right there; you think, "Oh no, not this again." But you live with it.

A fear of breast cancer, then, is not necessarily linked directly to experience of illness or the physical manifestations of illness such as a tumor. As Toombs shows, it is what these experiences might represent that invokes fear. For example, she states that it is an awareness that illness is capable of intruding upon everyday life that makes one fearful; illness represents the possible "impossibility of taking a walk around the block" and other such activities (Toombs, 1995, 10). Fear means recognizing the possibility that one's experiences of body may become restricted. It is a feeling that alters experiences of both embodiment and time, as one knows one's body in view of past, present, and future.

Fear also evolves within a particular social context, one in which bodies may be viewed as vehicles of social control. Kleinman states that "cancer seems to implicate our very way of life: what we choose to eat, what we like to do" (1988, 21). All causes of cancer are unknown, yet the predominant discourse suggests it is caused by individual inattention to diet or exercise. Diane may have indicated awareness of this discourse when she talked about what changes she was willing to make to her lifestyle after breast cancer. Paradoxically, when the sociocultural context of cancer is acknowledged discursively, it occurs in ways that suggest that it is "caused by everything and is everywhere" (Clarke, 1999, 119). Taken together, the individual emphases on cause/cure, along with a discourse of prevalence/uncertainty, imply that a fear of cancer, or its recurrence, is best understood phenomenologically. A phenomenological approach allows for an understanding of the intersubjective nature of experiences such as fear, and its relationship to particular social contexts.

EFFICACY OF PHENOMENOLOGY FOR RESEARCHING ILLNESS

The women I interviewed showed why it is important to understand the intersection of body and culture and how this intersection is representative of a fundamental betrayal of what they had taken for granted. These women illustrate much about the social construction of disability and what it might mean for them to be unable to do things that they once took for granted. They demonstrate that biomedical knowledge about fear of recurrence is limited. Yet these women direct attention to domains outside of breast cancer and illustrate the fragility of our world.

I believe that these women's words extend beyond their own experiences and express some of the uncertainty that people in general can feel in the face of individualistic prescriptions for avoiding illnesses such as cancer. Larger uncertainties, anxieties, and fears connect to society's limited but foreboding awareness of the potential impact of industrialization, environmental contamination, and degradation. A phenomenological study that captures women's experiences in their own words can provide an opportunity to understand something about the intersubjective nature of being.

The work of Husserl, Heidegger, and Merleau-Ponty facilitates the creation of critical knowledge that enables one to question those ontologies, epistemologies, and "the rule of the older natural sciences," which rarely recognize serious illness as a lifelong process (Watson, 1988, 15). In terms of the body, nursing scholars recognize that qualitative inquiry invites us to understand that "the lived world . . . is imbued with esthetic, moral, and personal meanings. Holistic nursing embodies these meanings as an integral aspect, rather than additions to nursing care" (Bishop and Scudder, 1997, ¶26; see also Watson, 1988). A phenomenological orientation to research is very much congruent with my interest in how illness becomes woven into the fabric of existence, in ways not readily understood through positivistic approaches. Phenomenology has also provided me with an opportunity to see how my sociological training in understanding inequality can be coupled with an understanding of individuals' experiences.

TRANSFORMATIONAL MOMENTS: FOR ME, FOR HEALTHCARE PRACTITIONERS, FOR PHYSICIANS

Broadly, healthcare practitioners increasingly recognize that the impact of cancer may be felt well beyond the conclusion of treatment for disease. However, phenomenological research demonstrates the current inadequacies of Western medicine as currently structured. Women with breast cancer have few, if any, opportunities to make sense of their experiences, particularly once they leave the realm of acute care. For instance, there is no national cancer rehabilitation program in Canada, despite the complex legacy of illness and treatment, which leaves cancer survivors grappling with many issues connected to embodiment, at the intersection of the physical and the social aspects of existence.

More specifically, clinical studies of cancer survivorship clearly demonstrate their limitations, with their emphases upon measuring human experience solely according to psychological scales. What the women in my study show is that fear of recurrence is incredibly complex and not easily reduced to a numerical score. For me, this clearly demonstrates the ways in which people who are ill may become marginalized through their encounters with biomedical practices, and the potential of phenomenology for understanding enigmatic experiences such as the fear of breast cancer recurrence.

There are also many significant implications for healthcare practitioners. How might a physician best respond to and support a woman who has experienced breast cancer? There is no prescribed treatment for the fear or complex array of emotions that follow this illness and its treatment. While the women in this study indicated that talking about their experiences with me was positive, it would be difficult, within the current confines of our healthcare system, to allow for the type of active listening associated with phenomenological research approaches to occur. Yet developing this role of the active listener could be valuable, not only for those with breast cancer, but also for those who experience other forms of chronic illness. Further, physicians themselves report their occupation as stressful; fulfilling such a role could make medical practice more meaningful, as has been my experience with teaching.

Since completing the study described in this chapter, I have been responsible for teaching several university-level courses in research methods. Many students have arrived in my classes with a high level of fear and anxiety, convinced that they cannot do research. Actively and openly listening to these fears has helped me to think about the ways in which I might positively approach the topic of research. Intentionally, I begin courses with phenomenological texts that are very much grounded in the authors' lives. Students are also encouraged to develop oral presentation skills, and are asked to think about how they listen and convey respect for ideas shared by others. Students see firsthand that research is not abstracted from life, in the same ways that healthcare practitioners might approach the complexity involved with understanding the patient's lifeworld as it is affected by illness.

Phenomenology may, therefore, act as an antidote to biomedical approaches that separate body and mind into dualistic categories. While I do see developing an understanding of fear as an essential aspect of healing for individuals, phenomenologically embracing embodiment as the intersection of body, mind, and society may mean that understanding and acknowledging fear more generally is a task for us all.

REFERENCES

Bentz, Valerie M., and Jeremy J. Shapiro. (1998) *Mindful Inquiry in Social Research.* Thousand Oaks, CA: Sage.

Bishop, Anne H., and John R. Scudder Jr. (1997) A Phenomenological Interpretation of Holistic Nursing. *Journal of Holistic Nursing, 15*(2), 103. Retrieved September 21, 1999, from http://www.ehostweb7.com/ehost1.asp.

Bordo, Susan. (1993) Postmodern Subjects, Postmodern Bodies, Postmodern Resistance. In S. Bordo (Ed.), *Unbearable Weight: Feminism, Western Culture, and the Body* (277–300). Berkeley: University of California Press.

Clarke, Juanne N. (1999) Breast Cancer in Mass Circulating Magazines in the U.S.A. and Canada, 1974–1995. *Women and Health, 28*(4), 113–30.

Gatens, Moira. (1996) *Imaginary Bodies: Ethics, Power and Corporeality.* New York: Routledge.

Hawkins, Joyce M. (Ed.). (1987) *The Oxford Paperback Dictionary.* Oxford: Oxford University Press.

Kleinman, Arthur. (1988) *The Illness Narratives: Suffering, Healing and the Human Condition.* New York: Basic Books.

Leder, Drew. (1990) Flesh and Blood: A Proposed Supplement to Merleau-Ponty. *Human Studies, 13*(3), 209–19.

———. (1992a) Introduction. In D. Leder (Ed.), *The Body in Medical Thought and Practice* (1–12). Dordrecht, The Netherlands: Kluwer Academic.

———. (1992b) A Tale of Two Bodies: The Cartesian Corpse and the Lived Body. In D. Leder, (Ed.), *The Body in Medical Thought and Practice* (17–35). Dordrecht, The Netherlands: Kluwer Academic.

Mathieson, Cynthia. (1994) Women with Cancer and the Meaning of Body Talk. *Canadian Woman Studies, 14*(3), 52–55.

Merleau-Ponty, Maurice. (1962) *Phenomenology of Perception.* (C. Smith, Trans.) New York: The Humanities Press.

Munhall, Patricia L. (1994) *Revisioning Phenomenology: Nursing and Health Science.* New York: National League for Nursing.

Olesen, Virginia L. (1992) Extraordinary Events and Mundane Ailments: The Contextual Dialectics of the Embodied Self. In Carolyn Ellis and Michael G. Flaherty (Eds.), *Investigating Subjectivity: Research on Lived Experience* (205–20). Newbury Park, CA: Sage.

Rehorick, David A. (1986) Shaking the Foundations of Lifeworld: A Phenomenological Account of an Earthquake Experience. *Human Studies, 9,* 379–91.

Thomas, Roanne. (1994) *"Cancer is . . .?" An Exploration of Adults' Accounts of Living with Cancer.* Unpublished MA Thesis. Fredericton, Canada: University of New Brunswick.

Toombs, S. Kay. (1992) *The Meaning of Illness: A Phenomenological Account of the Different Perspectives of Physician and Patient.* Dordrecht, The Netherlands: Kluwer.

———. (1995) The Lived Experience of Disability. *Human Studies, 18,* 9–23.

van Manen, Max. (1998) Modalities of Body Experience in Illness and Health. *Qualitative Health Research, 8*(1), 7. Retrieved September 23, 1999, from http://www.ehostweb7.com/ehost1.asp.

Watson, Jean. (1988) *Nursing: Human Science and Human Care. A Theory of Nursing.* New York: National League for Nursing.

6

Take My Kidney Please

An Organ Donor's Experience

Jeffrey L. Nonemaker

NOVEMBER 25, 1997, LAIKON HOSPITAL, ATHENS, GREECE

My calmness frightens me. This fact should be registering in the audible, electronic throb of my monitored heartbeat. But it's pulsing on steadily and slowly, punctuating the whir of the room's air conditioning.

I try to slow the rhythm further by mentally playing with the beat for a few minutes, thinking about the sea in summer.

this must be the ultimate biofeedback machine. . . .

My thoughts are here and everywhere.

probably from the Demerol . . .

"Einai ksenos?" (Is he a foreigner?) asks someone from somewhere in the room.

"Malista." (Yes.) "Emai Amerikanos." (I'm an American.)

my speech is slurred. . . .

A woman with smiling eyes above her masked mouth appears, partially blocking the huge light fixture that hangs above me.

"From which state?" she asks, challenging my flawed Greek.

"California."

"I've been to Los Angeles and San Francisco!" she comments cheerfully, as I feel yet another needle being set into my forearm.

From some corner of the room, I hear, "Pios nefro; dexia, h aristera?" (Which kidney; right, or left?) The question bounces off the high-gloss, green walls.

"Aristera!" (Left) I say, too loudly.

For God's sake, I hope they take the correct one.

"Do you understand Greek?" another masked face asks.

"Malista," (Yes) I answer.

"Is the recipient your brother?" He continues in English anyway.

"No . . . a colleague."

"Po, po!" (My, my!) "He must be a *very* good colleague for you to give such a gift!"

Trying desperately to think about his statement, I realize that I'm lying here naked, cold, strapped down, spread cruciform, and tethered to a dozen machines by tubes and wires, waiting for the surgeons to remove a healthy organ of mine and place it into another body, my colleague's body, Dimitri.

AUGUST, 1996, NEA MAKRI, GREECE

Even though the cool Aegean was visible from the courtyard of the cemetery's chapel, its proximity did nothing to stop the perspiration that was soaking my shirt and underclothing beneath my black suit. The sun had once again unmercifully turned the plane of Marathon into a sweltering patchwork of olive groves, farms, and dwellings. I, out of respect and duty, was a reluctant element of that pattern. An August afternoon is not the most convenient time for a funeral, I thought to myself, but then death never seems to be cognizant of convenience. I was glad to have been able to quit the chapel's small, stifling interior at the end of the liturgy. Though I had been standing there in honor and tribute to a colleague who had been killed in a tragic automobile accident, I was distracted by the discomfort caused by the crush of bodies, the fog of incense, and the droning of the priest.

Once I was outside the chapel, a hot, late afternoon breeze disturbed the rhythm of the cicadas chanting in the pines, but did not deter the priests' continuing song as the casket-enclosed body was placed into the waiting hearse. The priests ended the Orthodox ceremony, and then someone began a eulogy in English. The speaker paused, for a moment, and a familiar voice, echoing the words in their Greek translation, caused me to look up; it was Dimitri. I had not seen him since the academic term had ended last June. He looked dreadful. His illness had not allowed him to spend his normal summer idyll on the island of Tilos. Instead, he had been bound to the routine of dialysis, clinic visits, and the unnerving, polluted heat and traffic of Athens.

"Dear God," I thought. "Will he be the next one we'll bury?"

A SOLITARY STRUGGLE: SHOULD I DONATE A KIDNEY?

I, Jeff, the donor, am a fifty-seven-year-old, male Caucasian. I live with Patti, my wife and friend of thirty-five years, in a northern suburb of Athens, Greece. Our two children, Gretchen and Aaron, are grown and out of the nest, now residing in the United States. As a baby boomer, weaned on life in Southern California in the 1950s, I matured within that unique culture and became a veteran of the 1960s and, ultimately, the Vietnam War. In the 1970s, I enjoyed all the accoutrements of a fast-track professional, until I bailed out in search of an adventure and moved my then-young family to Greece in 1983.

In 1994, I had come to a point in my life where I stopped to assess how much I had been given (or had taken). I summarized my life in these terms:

> I have enjoyed the comforts of wealth, and have known the misery of poverty. I have grasped babies crying and kicking from the womb, and have held men as they drew their last breath. I have known the indescribable joys of love, and the unspeakable void of loneliness. I have visited some of the most beautiful places on this planet, and the most devastated. I have partaken of the fruits of peace, and have experienced the hell of war. I have had the freedom to create, and the freedom to destroy. I have known the Grace of God, and have flirted with the devil.

Dimitri, the recipient, was born in Patras, Greece, in 1943, the first son of a prominent banker. He spent his formative years in post–civil war Greece until he traveled to the United States as a high school exchange student with the American Field Service in 1961. Drawn to American culture and the academy, he completed an undergraduate degree at CUNY in 1966 and then his graduate and Ph.D. degrees at Columbia in 1972. Returning to Greece, he began his professional life as a sociology professor and researcher. Over the years, his distinctive senses of humor and charm have endeared him to his students and colleagues. One particular student, a talented, classically trained dancer named Lily, was charmed enough to marry him.

I met Dimitri in 1983, when I took on an academic administrative position at an American university's overseas campus in Athens. He was a member of my faculty. In this academic relationship, we often did not see eye to eye, but had developed a mutual respect for one another over the years.

Dimitri suffered from varying effects of high blood pressure for several years. Unfortunately, his physicians failed to check the state of his kidneys during his treatment for hypertension and prescribed medication that eventually led to kidney dysfunction. After a series of medical emergencies, he underwent a renal biopsy. It was then that Dimitri was diagnosed as suffering from IgA Nephropathy (IgAN), a disease that damages the tiny filtering structures of the kidney and diminishes function. His loss of kidney function quickly progressed to chronic kidney failure and end-stage renal disease. This required hemodialysis treatment; ultimately, he needed a kidney transplant to maintain life. Unfortunately, there is a dearth of available donor kidneys in Greece.

An interview recorded in 2000 on a Greek public television documentary regarding the transplantation question in Greece highlighted this desperate situation:

> *Commentator:* Being the director of the dialysis unit in Laiko Hospital [Athens, Greece], you are aware of the magnitude of the problem for both the people who are on dialysis and the acute problem regarding transplantations in Greece.
>
> *Dialysis Unit Director:* We are one of the last countries, the last country in Europe, in [number of] transplantations.
>
> *Commentator:* In the country that is number 1 in vehicle accident fatalities [per capita in Europe]?
>
> *Dialysis Unit Director:* In most countries, there are twenty to sixty transplantations per one million people annually. In Greece, this number is approximately eight per million population. Nationally, our patients on dialysis number 7,500! There is, therefore, an acute problem regarding kidney supply. (Laskari, 2000)

Dimitri's deteriorating health, and the regime of three four-hour dialysis treatments per week, caused his life and lifestyle to be inexorably changed. By 1996, the once-happy and fulfilled individual had become disconsolate, and terminally ill.

NOVEMBER, 1996, ST. ANDREW'S CHURCH, ATHENS, GREECE

It was Sunday and Advent. I sat listening to a sermon about giving; it was a fitting subject for the holiday season. During the sermon, the minister used an illustration from a news article involving two retired California men who happen to meet while fishing on a local pier. His story unfolded this way:

> The men casually greeted one another and settled into the business of preparing their fishing tackle. As custom would have it, one man asked the other how he was doing.
>
> "I'm not doing so well," the man replied. "I'm very tired and kind of depressed, I guess, because of a long illness."
>
> "What's wrong with you?" the other asked.
>
> "My kidneys have quit working, I'm on dialysis, and things don't look too good for me. I'm one of 40,000 other people in the States waiting for a transplant."
>
> "Why are they waiting?"
>
> "For a kidney to be donated!" he replied, a little irritated at the man's stupidity.
>
> They enjoyed one another's company and made arrangements to meet the next day.

During the next visit, after sitting together and fishing in silence, one man casually said to the other, "I've got two kidneys, and I only need one. Do you want one of mine?" ("A Gift to a Stranger," 1991)

Over the next two months, the minister's illustration and my thoughts of Dimitri's illness returned to me at least once a day. Their annoying, frequent recurrence caused me to reexamine my beliefs more closely. I would turn the thought of my involvement carefully in my mind, as I would if I were holding an unidentifiable, possibly dangerous object in my hands. Where did the idea come from? What's the use of such ponderings? Will the contemplation of action harm me? Whatever possessed me to examine the idea in the first place?

There were days when I would feel this tremendous pressure to do something with these burdensome thoughts—write about them, tell someone about them—but to do so would have been a kind of conscious acknowledgment of their weight. If I didn't tell anyone what I was thinking, no one would be disappointed if I ended up making a wrong choice. I wanted to tell Patti about this, but how was I going to explain this to her, when I couldn't figure it out myself?

Okay, here's how it might go: "Hi babe! How was your day? Mine? Oh, the usual. . . . I survived another faculty meeting. Then, in the afternoon, I decided to give one of my kidneys to Dimitri." (That won't play!)

Before I burdened her with my contemplation of this decision, I wanted to be more certain that it was a *real* possibility. My hesitation wasn't borne out of fear of her reaction, but rather it was out of the sureness of our love. We've shared our lives for over thirty years, and I knew that the wisdom we've gained from this would move her beyond any uncertainties she might have. When the time came that I felt I had enough information to allow me to talk with her about the possibility of my being a donor, I knew that she would enclose us in her faith and love, and honor whatever decision I made. Moore suggested that "the point of marriage is not to create a material, human world, but rather to evoke a spirit of love that is not of this world" (1994, 52). My knowledge of Patti and our life experiences as a couple assured me that such a spirit existed in our relationship. She would understand my initial hesitation because she loved and understood me completely.

This assurance didn't lessen the fact that I wanted to forget about these uncomfortable promptings. And I still hoped that Dimitri's illness would be taken care of without me. That didn't happen. I would see Dimitri or hear someone mention his name, and the question would pose itself again: "What are *you* going to do?"

SEARCHING FOR FIRST-PERSON VOICE:
PHENOMENOLOGY AND AUTOETHNOGRAPHY

I digress from my account to discuss how this work came into being. I wanted to use my experience of becoming a kidney donor as the topic of my doctoral dissertation. The primary data for the study was my personal journals. Other important sources included audiotaped conversations and written text provided by Dimitri, his family, and my own immediate family. All were asked to build upon my text. Translated texts from Greek newspaper and periodical articles about the transplant and translated transcriptions of segments from two Greek television news features and a television documentary were also included.

As the data from these different sources began to accumulate, I realized that I was beginning to have difficulty with formatting the narrative. The polyvocality of the participants that was emerging was demanding something other than a traditional writing form (Gergen and Gergen, 2000; Green, 2000; Lincoln and Denzin, 1994). My initial writings about being a potential donor were mostly seat-of-the-pants stuff born of intuition.

I found methodological pathways through phenomenology, autoethnography, and other qualitative approaches. Phenomenology, particularly that of Clark Moustakas, guided my search for patterns and relationships leading to enhanced meanings, and deepened and extended my knowledge (1990, 24). Autoethnography encouraged me to produce a text that, as Carolyn Ellis suggests,

> celebrates concrete experience and intimate detail; examines how human experience is endowed with meaning; is concerned with moral, ethical and political consequences; encourages compassion and empathy; helps us to know how to live and cope; features multiple voices and repositions the readers and subjects as co-participants in dialogue; seeks a fusion between social science and literature and connects the practices of social science with the living of life. (1999, 669)

Such a view of theory and writing contests traditional standards for undertaking scholarly research and inquiry. One result of this is the meeting of previously separated methods of research and methods of expression (Langellier, 1989). Evoking emotional responses to symbolic experience through personal narratives (Denzin, 1999; Ellis, 2000), questioning the conventions and parameters of science (Richardson, 2000; Tierney and Lincoln, 1997), and intertwining the personal and the professional (Ellis, 1999) are among recent objectives that have been identified and explored through text. It is this accounting for and full employment of the researcher's personal body and felt experience that has led to the development and rise of *autoethnography* (see Clough, 1997; Ellis, 1999; Plummer,

1999; Richardson, 1999). Autoethnography is an autobiographical genre of writing and research that displays multiple layers of consciousness, connecting the personal with the cultural. Usually written in first-person voice, autoethnographic texts appear in a variety of forms (Ellis, 2000, 739).

The kindred methodological natures of phenomenology and autoethnography, with their emphasis on first-person descriptive accounts, offered a way to capture my experience of kidney donation. Max van Manen explicates clearly the place of first-person accounts in phenomenological inquiry (1997, 2002).

HERMENEUTIC UNDERSTANDINGS: BUILDING AN INFORMED KNOWLEDGE BASE

"Organ donation." No, worse: "*Living* organ donation." I didn't even like the sound of the phrase! These words belonged in someone else's lexicon, *not* mine. So why was I plagued by thoughts of personal involvement in such an act?

I realized that one of the reasons I was having difficulty putting this question behind me was that I was ill-informed about transplant surgery. I could generally locate the kidneys in a human being. Although I basically knew their function, I hadn't a clue about kidney disease, kidney transplants, or living organ donation. I found online links to organizations, newsgroups, and support groups that dealt with facts, statistics, and issues about organ transplantation. As my knowledge of kidney disease and the statistical information regarding renal transplantation increased, the ever-present question remained: "Could I *really* offer my kidney to Dimitri?"

After some time, I realized that I didn't necessarily want to know about specific medical information, but I did want to understand: "What *exactly* happens to one's body during live organ transplantation?" I understood from my previous research that the answer was probably (in all too graphic format) available online for me to access. So I sampled from a staggering array of data. I viewed all the details through the barely open fingers of my hands that covered my face. I even found photographs and videos of the transplant procedure. Despite my discomfort, I continued my research, focusing next on what happens at an institutional level.

Working from Greece, I relied heavily upon information and resources available through the Internet. This enabled me to define the scope of the medical and related social environments of organ donation and transplantation. Toward the end of my search, I found, quite by accident, a link to TransWeb, and roamed its wide and sometimes too vivid, donor-friendly halls (Regents of the University of Michigan, 2003). In one prominent section entitled *Real People*, I discovered a listing of narratives that living donors had posted about their transplant experiences. The first one I read was subtitled *Experiences of a Male Living Kidney Donor*. It began:

> I've found that there are very few fence-sitters out there when it comes to the decision to donate a kidney: either you've already decided you will and are afraid of what you'll find here, or you've decided you don't want to and are looking for reasons to support your decision. This is not about why to donate; that's up to you. (Glazewski, 1999, 1)

This story, written in a straightforward and self-effacing manner, was the beginning of a quantum leap toward my knowing what living organ donation encompassed. I immediately read the thirty others that were posted, and then began to follow links to other sites containing donors' stories. I read voraciously and reread each story that I located, mentally cataloguing every detail. My preconceived understanding and concepts about being a living donor were challenged. As Norman Denzin contends, I was moving swiftly in that hermeneutic circle where interpretation both unravels what is understood and produces understanding. Understanding, in turn, rewrites interpretation (1989, 252).

Upon further reflection, I understood that the *events*, not the stories created about these acts, were commanding my attention. The styles of the stories were merely transparent modes, unambiguously reflecting stable, multiple meanings. Their rootedness in time, place, and personal experience, in their perspective-ridden character, rendered the stories of value to me (Riessman, 1993, 4). These personal experience narratives also made meaning through the common understandings and language existing among living organ donors. As simple as many of the narratives were, they spoke directly to me with authenticity and clarity.

Interpretation is transformative, Denzin advocates. It illuminates and throws light on the experience. It brings out and refines the meanings that can be sifted from a text or a slice of an experience (1994, 504). Transformed and illuminated by my engagement with these stories, I wondered if the key to understanding how to proceed toward making my decision might lie in pursuing a similar writing process (see Brooks, 1984; Bruner, 1987). I revisited the narratives, where I found allusions to and comments about fear for the body. All the donors had placed themselves on the dangerous edge, believing that their decisions were right ones, even though death was a possible outcome. I put aside the narratives for a time in order to digest this information.

Days later, I returned to my notes and found that the data had not magically changed in my absence. I had to face what was evident. Fear was the core of my own discomfort. My fear was real. Fear had put me in an inauthentic state. Borders that had distinguished my personal confidence were disappearing as I contemplated my donation decision. Martin Heidegger notes that fear is fearing in the face of a threatening force that draws near (1927/1964, 179–82). Not only was the point of resolution out there, but the *consequences* of my choice were also moving toward me with unknown speed and force. An empty-handed feeling of defenselessness dominated my mind.

Fear was located *in* my body, and there was fear *for* my body: my instrument in the world that makes me visible and accessible to the doings, accomplishments, and gazes of others (Denzin, 1989, 87). I did *not* want my body to become less accessible to the world, repugnant in the gaze of others, nor, most of all, to cease being. When circumstances force us to acknowledge death's relationship to ourselves, we tend to think it is something that *will* happen (Heidegger, 1927/1964, 280–81). Though death is always present, we do not know what to do with the issues about mortality. I did not want to force the relationship before its time.

I paused and studied the list of my fears again. The words created a visual and cognitive, rough harmony, faceted with a potential for multilayered interconnections. I rewrote and rearranged my fears in lines and columns, in variations and scatterations, drew connecting arrows, added notes, ideas, and brief reflections. This tentative, initial writing exercise had been an act of discovery, revealing the truth of my fear and anxiety (see Kierkegaard, 1844/1957). My aim was to organize and interpret the reality of my personal experience in a way that would mesh with and add new meaning to the deep structures of existing donor narratives, and inform and create knowledge for the organ transplantation community (donors, recipients, medical teams) and the greater public. In addition to this task of writing it up would be the crucial challenge of balancing, harmonizing, mediating, and otherwise negotiating a tale of two cultures—Greek and expatriate American.

Telling stories in postmodern times attempts to change one's own life by affecting the lives of others (Frank, 1995, 18). It was within the spirit of this statement that I proceeded. Not only did I have a story to tell, I had to tell Dimitri, somehow, that *we* had a story. After two months of reflection and research, I knew that it was *possible* for me to be his donor.

TELLING DIMITRI: A PHENOMENOLOGICAL ACCOUNT

Thursday morning, February 20, 1997, Dimitri arrived in my office, and we began our meeting with some normal academic business. I got up and made an excuse to close my door, citing the noise from some construction activity in the building as distracting. As I walked back to my desk, I could feel my pulse racing and the dryness in my throat as I swallowed. I settled into my chair as best I could, given the tenseness of my body at that moment.

"How are you holding up Dimitri?"

"To tell you the truth, Jeff, with great difficulty, but I'm strong."

I was trying to listen carefully to his every word, because he was describing a reality of which I might soon be a part. Thinking back, though, I can't remember much of what he specifically said; I was too full of thoughts about my own words that I was finally going to verbalize. He paused for a moment, and I jumped in with both feet.

"Dimitri, there's something that I've been wanting to say to you, but I've been afraid of saying it out of my own fear, and out of the fear that you will think it's just some altruistic baloney."

"Come on . . ." he protested, as if what was coming was going to be an embarrassment to him.

"Dimitri, I have two good kidneys: one for me and one for you." My voice shook.

There was a shock of silence, both too loud and too quiet.

"Asta!" (Leave it!) "Jeff . . . please . . ." he finally was able to say. He wanted me to stop.

"Please, listen to me, Dimitri. Over the past few years, I have spent a lot of time examining who I am, why I am, and what I'm all about. And you know what? I have come to the pleasant conclusion that I like who I am, and have had the privilege of living quite an exceptional life. In fact, if the proverbial lightning bolt struck me at this very moment and I died, I would leave this earth smiling, and . . ."

"Give me your hand," he interrupted, leaning forward and extending his own hand across my desk.

"Come on; I'm serious . . . !"

"Jeff," he laughed, shaking his head, "How is it that you can be so impossible at times as the dean, and then say something like this?"

"I think possibly deans are human, Dimitri." I paused a moment to collect myself, and then continued. "Dimitri, I have been given so much in my life. Please, allow me to give you something of myself," I said, grasping his proffered hand.

"Jeff, I'm sincerely moved by this . . . but, to be honest, I don't think I have the strength to be moved today!" He smiled and continued. "Other people have said the same kind of things to me."

I felt that he hadn't taken my words seriously, that they were just another sympathetic expression to him. "I'm serious, Dimitri! I want to be a donor for you. I still have a lot of questions about it, but if I'm a near match for you, I'll do it."

Laughing, he formed an embarrassed smile. "We'll talk about it. Let's leave it for today." He started to change the subject, to fake me out. Then, characteristically, he abruptly looked me directly in the eyes with a crazy grin and quickly asked, "What's your blood type?"

"O positive."

"That's the right one!"

We spent a few minutes sharing our collective ignorance about tissue typing, cross-matching, and blood work, and about his chances of receiving a kidney from a cadaveric source. Then, he invited me to come to visit him during one of his dialysis sessions at the clinic that week.

"That will be a real eye opener for you. You've never seen anything like it!"

I told him I'd try to make it to the hospital at his convenience.

"I have a class I need to get to," he said as he stood and gathered up his coat and brief case.

"Dimitri, I'd appreciate it if you didn't share this conversation with anyone. I don't think it's necessary to go public with this."

"Of course!" he replied. "Do you mind if I tell Lily?"

"No, that would be fine. I'm not going to share this with Patti, though, until I know some more about it." I came around my desk to say goodbye and open the door for him. I offered my hand, and he took it and pulled me toward him.

"Come here." He put his arms around me and hugged me tightly. Kissing me on both cheeks, he said simply, "Thanks, I sincerely am moved by this."

As he left my office, I knew without a doubt that neither our relationship nor our lives would ever be the same.

The next day, his wife Lily, who teaches dance for the university, stopped by before her class. "Hi Jeff; how are you? Dimitri wanted me to give this to you." She seemed nervous and a little distracted as she handed me an envelope. We spent a few moments talking about banal matters before she hurriedly left. I sat down, opened the envelope and took out the note. It read:

> Jeff: All I want to tell you is that
>
> your thoughts on the issue we discussed
>
> yesterday represent for me the ultimate one
>
> can extend to another human. I will not
>
> forget it, ever.
>
>   Dimitri C.

I felt as if something had suddenly gripped my heart and consciousness and thought:

"My God! What have I done?"

The moment that I read Dimitri's note, I understood that I had moved beyond the theoretical, "*What if?*" stage and into a different reality. I had, by my actions and words, placed myself in a world that I had not foreseen as existing, let alone one to be experiencing. The phenomenon of "*What now?*" was in dire need of dialogue in order for me to understand its creation and meaning.

We experience our world as differentiated phenomenologically, yet we cannot contemplate many of its differentiations cognitively—cannot see *itself* in itself—because we lack concepts for them. This particular phenomenon was far beyond any of my known personal concepts. If, however, we can first identify these phenomenological units at the edge of our awareness, and then point out the experiential boundaries around them that cut off one phenomenon from another, we can begin to supply the concepts that allow this contemplation. At this point, the only concept that I could contemplate was adventure, but one entirely unique to my experience. The beginning of this adventure had been astonishing to me. Not knowing its possible content or ending was causing me a good deal of personal anxiety. Though comfortable with the physical boundaries of personally known social phenomena, I could not yet imagine, nor did I want to encounter, the phenomenological boundaries and depths of this experience.

With this beginning, I would have to trust that the mechanisms that would navigate me to and through the encounter were within me, or obtainable along the way. As the arbitrator of my own presence in the world, I would have the last word on this adventure.

What had I done? Making meaning of this question, and the adventure of the encounter ahead, might lie in an hermeneutic cycle of returning and reflecting on the question itself, a spiral of guess and validation, and a continual resetting of boundaries (Bentz and Shapiro, 1998, 112).

RE-VOICING THE TRANSPLANT EXPERIENCE:
A PERPETUAL NOW

Nearly twelve months elapsed from the day I first began to *think* about being Dimitri's donor until the transplant took place. The majority of this time was spent trying to convince the chief of the transplant unit of the Greek state hospital that the operation could and *should* take place. This doctor, the head of our potential surgical team, was fully aware that the removal and transfer of an organ from a living, unrelated donor to another person was ethically and legally not without problems or controversy in Greece. From 1990 to 1996, he and his surgical teams performed at least half of the 238 living donor kidney transplants in Greece. More than 90 percent had involved genetically or emotionally related donors; the remainder involving cadaveric donations. *Related—that* was the key to the medical establishment's suspicion and the source of my frustration. I was the anomaly. I was the factor that did not figure in the Greek solution of the transplant equation. I had made an unsolicited offer as an unrelated donor. At that time, there was no history or precedent for dealing with this. My offer and presence were a new twist in the Greek transplant equation. In addition to this, I was a foreigner. Or, as the doctor quite frankly put it to me, I was "a wise-ass American with an Internet connection that spits out nothing but bullshit information about transplants."

The other major complication arose from the fact that Dimitri and I were a zero-match histologically. None of six possible matches of antigens was present between us. A zero-match transplant had never been performed in Greece until 1996. However, I found evidence in medical journal articles that transplants had been performed successfully under such a condition in several other countries in recent years. I gave copies of these articles to the doctor; they were pronounced additional bullshit.

Ultimately, the doctor convinced Dimitri not to go through the danger of a transplant involving me. He promised Dimitri that he would deliver, within three months, a cadaveric kidney that would be a better match than I would be. Reluctantly, Dimitri agreed to wait, but, after weeks of legal wrangling, we secured an agreement from the doctor that if this did not happen, he would finally perform the surgery with me as the donor. To obtain this agreement, I had to sign publicly a legal document that would absolve the doctor from all responsibility if any problems or deaths resulted. As I had expected, the promised cadaveric kidney did not materialize after three months, and our transplant was finally scheduled.

NOVEMBER 25, 1997, ST. CATHERINE'S DAY

I was awakened early and given an injection. "This will help you rest," said the nurse. As soon as she left, there was a knock on the door, and Dimitri came in to wish me well. But we were only able to exchange a few brief, emotional sentences before orderlies came in to take me away to the surgical theater.

Ceilings and light fixtures dizzily move by overhead. Strangers inquisitively peer down at me, hoping to guess my condition and fate, many of them automatically crossing themselves in the Greek Orthodox fashion. The gurney turns again, and I'm propelled into a wide passageway in which I hear familiar voices. The concerned but smiling faces of my wife and friends pass over me, moments before we noisily break through swinging doors and enter a cool, dark hallway. I feel the gurney suddenly halt, and hear its brake snap into place.

"Perimenoumae," (we wait here) the orderly casually says, then disappears.

Suddenly, I'm moving again through more doors into a colder, larger space: the operating theater. Once transferred on to the operating table, I'm strapped down, and quickly surrounded by green-clad technicians. In the midst of my slurred banter in Greek and English, I am pierced too many times and connected to countless machines and monitors.

"Mr. Jeffrey!" Two hands cradle my head; the upside-down face of the anaesthesiologist comes into view over me. "We're just about ready to begin. How do you feel?"

"Just breathe normally, please." He places the plastic mask over my nose and mouth.

I move my eyes to the digital clock pulsing its blood-red display. My heartbeat, coming from a great distance now, is a little slower than the passing of time. I trace along the wall to an exposed corner of a curtained window. There are raindrops on the glass.

I want to close my eyes. Nothing would feel better right now. I need to close my eyes and think about the process and reasoning that brought me to be lying here, prepped, and draped in green linen.

"Mr. Jeffrey, Mr. Jeffrey! It's time to wake up! Everything went beautifully. Your kidney is already making your friend well! Mr. Jeffrey, open your eyes! Your surgery is finished. The doctors are just finishing with your friend. Mr. Jeffrey, wake up now! Please, open your eyes! They'll be taking you back to your room in just a few minutes."

I don't want to open my eyes all the way yet. I'll just crack them a bit and take in what I can. The clock, someone has messed with it, or I'm not reading the numbers correctly. Seven hours have passed since I last glanced at it.

"I'm freezing," I croak.

I can't hear my heartbeat any longer. Am I dead?

Now the ceiling is flying by too rapidly. The phenomenon and the movement of the gurney make me woozy.

"There he is!" a familiar voice calls out.

Straining to focus my eyes, I see Patti standing in the hallway ahead. I lift a tube-implanted hand and wave to them as I pass.

"How's Dimitri doing?" someone calls out as I roll by.

The gurney makes several sharp turns, then stops. Surrounded by muffled voices (angels?!), I momentarily feel body and soul float upward before gravity mercifully pulls me down again. They secure me to earth with snug sheets and plastic tubes.

The routines and schedule of the transplant ward quickly established themselves. Each night, I was watched over and cared for by my nurse, and by day, my wife was there, seeing to my needs in so many ways and organizing the seemingly endless parade of visitors and well-wishers. I felt a little stronger, and could move myself about more freely, each day. Dimitri's condition continued to improve dramatically. The transplant that the doctor had warned us against had thus far been a success. Our daily post-op tests continued to yield good news. Within three days, Dimitri's new kidney had obliterated all toxins from his system.

RENEWED BODY AS OPENING TO THE TRANSPLANTED SELF

Ten years have passed since the day of the transplant. Dimitri remains in good health overall, and has now retired from his university teaching and research. During this period, he competed in two World Transplant Olympics and won gold medals in swimming and table tennis. I returned to the United States in 2005 and remain, to this day, active and very healthy. With each successive year, I'm more positive about the experience and grateful that the transplant has been such a success on many levels.

What *is*, then, the experience of giving the self as body? First, the question requires some additional qualifiers. Let's add, *What is (my) experience of giving (my) self as (my) body (in Greece), (in 1997)?* This version of the question is more descriptive of what my research and writing have revealed. My own transplantation encounter was a *total* experience, one involving all of the physical, cognitive, and psychological aspects of being. It is only now, years afterward, that I am able to understand the transplant's significance as a personally meaningful, transcendent experience (not unlike a religious one). Was it a hero's experience? Not in the classic sense. To call me a *hero* would be to deprive each of us of the responsibility for what we do and fail to do in our everyday lives as human mortals for one another.

Along the way, I saw a fellow human who was suffering and in need of assistance, and I stopped. Initially, I did *not* want to help; I was frightened by the thought of giving aid and what that aid might cost in terms of time and personal risk, quite unlike a hero's response. What finally prompted my action, and ultimately changed my life, was a simple call, much like T. S. Eliot's voice of the hidden waterfall, not known, because not looked for, but heard, half-heard, in the stillness (1963, 239), that asked, Who *is* my neighbor? The question itself sets a condition of complete simplicity. The very question is a divine gift of grace, a special, unwarranted favor that always requires a response. The gift of my self to Dimitri, wrapped in grace, reflected the spiraling way in which grace moves in the world: giving, receiving, and giving again. Brehony aptly called this ordinary grace:

> Our rational minds might ask why someone would undergo radical surgery, and the extraction of an organ from his or her own body, for a casual friend. When you look deeper, you see that in the cycle of grace, determining who has been giving and who has been receiving is not so easy. (1999, 84)

The realization of this idea may seem simplistic, but I've learned from the experience of giving self that ordinary grace occurs not only in giving one's body but also, and more importantly, in multitudes of small, daily actions, sometimes as simple as offering a kind word, or allowing someone to pull ahead of me in traffic. Ordinary grace loves the vernacular, the earthy, the present, and the real (119). It merely requires my attending and being open to opportunities.

I close this report of my personal experience and the research that emerged from it with an expanded sense of self, knowing that I have received a gift far more remarkable than that which I gave. If I *were* a hero or a saint, the boon that I would return to the world would be this simple truth that Arthur Frank wrote in 1995:

> If people could believe that each of us lacks something that only the other can fill—if we could be communicative bodies—then empathy would no longer be spoken as something that someone "has for" another. Instead, empathy is what a person "is with" another: a relationship in which each understands herself as requiring completion by the other. (150)

REFERENCES

A Gift to a Stranger: After 3-day Friendship, Fisherman Offered His Ailing Buddy a Kidney. (September 6, 1991) *Omaha World-Herald*, 38.

Bentz, Valerie M., and Jeremy J. Shapiro. (1998) *Mindful Inquiry in Social Research*. Thousand Oaks, CA: Sage.

Brehony, Kathleen. (1999) *Ordinary Grace*. New York: Riverhead.

Brooks, Peter. (1984) *Reading for the Plot: Design and Intention in Narrative*. Cambridge, MA: Harvard University Press.

Bruner, Jerome S. (1987) Life as Narrative. *Social Research, 54,* 11–22.

Clough, Patricia T. (1997) Autotelecommunication and Autoethnography: A Reading of Carolyn Ellis' Final Negotiations. *The Sociological Quarterly, 38,* 95–110.

Denzin, Norman K. (1989) *Interpretive Biography*. Thousand Oaks, CA: Sage.

———. (1994) *The Art and Politics of Interpretation*. In N. K. Denzin and Y. S. Lincoln (Eds.), *Handbook of Qualitative Research* (500–515). Thousand Oaks, CA: Sage.

———. (1999) Two-Stepping in the 90s. *Qualitative Inquiry, 5*(4), 568–72.

Eliot, Thomas S. (1963) *Collected Poems, 1909–1962*. New York: Harcourt, Brace Jovanovich.

Ellis, Carolyn. (1999) Heartful Autoethnography. *Qualitative Health Research, 9*(5), 669–83.

———. (2000). Creating Criteria: An Ethnographic Short Story. *Qualitative Inquiry, 6*(2), 273–77.

Frank, Arthur. (1995) *The Wounded Storyteller: Body, Illness and Ethics*. Chicago: University of Chicago Press.

Gergen, Mary, and Kenneth J. Gergen. (2000) Qualitative Inquiry: Tensions and Transformations. In N. K. Denzin and Y. S. Lincoln (Eds.), *Handbook of Qualitative Research* (second ed., 1025–46). Thousand Oaks, CA: Sage.

Glazewski, Stephen. *The Steve G Story: Experiences of a Male Living Kidney Donor*. Retrieved January 28, 2008, from http://www.transweb.org/people/live_don/experien/glazwski.htm.

Green, Jennifer C. (2000) Understanding Social Programs Through Evaluation. In N. K. Denzin and Y. S. Lincoln (Eds.), *Handbook of Qualitative Research* (second ed., 981–99). Thousand Oaks, CA: Sage.

Heidegger, Martin. (1927/1964) *Being and Time*. New York: Harper & Row.

Kierkegaard, Soren. (1844/1957) *The Concept of Dread* (W. Lowrie, Trans.) Princeton, NJ: Princeton University Press.

Langellier, Kristin. (1989) Personal Narratives: Perspectives on Theory and Research. *Text and Performance Quarterly*, 9, 243–76.

Laskari, Vicki (Executive Producer). (October 8, 2000) *Oso Iparhoun Anthropie* (As Long as There Are People). Athens: Hellenic Radio and Television 1 (ERT1).

Lincoln, Yvonna S., and Norman K. Denzin. (1994) The Fifth Movement. In N. K. Denzin and Y. S. Lincoln (Eds.), *Handbook of Qualitative Research* (575–86). Thousand Oaks, CA: Sage.

Moore, Thomas. (1994) *Soul Mates: Honoring the Mysteries of Love and Relationship*. New York: HarperPerennial.

Moustakas, Clark. (1990) *Heuristic Research: Design, Methodology, and Applications*. Newbury Park, CA: Sage.

Plummer, Ken. (1999) The "Ethnographic Society" at Century's End. *Journal of Contemporary Ethnography*, 28(6), 641–49.

Regents of the University of Michigan. (2003) *About TransWeb*. Retrieved January 28, 2008, from http://www.transweb.org/about_tw/about_tw.htm.

Riessman, Catherine. (1993) *Narrative Analysis*. Newbury Park, CA: Sage.

Richardson, Laurel. (1999) Feathers in our Cap. *Journal of Contemporary Ethnography*, 28(6), 660–68.

———. (2000). Writing: A Method of Inquiry. In N. K. Denzin and Y. S. Lincoln (Eds.), *Handbook of Qualitative Research* (second ed., 923–48). Thousand Oaks, CA: Sage.

Tierney, William G., and Yvonna S. Lincoln (Eds.). (1997) *Representation and the Text: Reframing the Narrative Voice*. Albany: State University of New York Press.

van Manen, Max. (1997). *Researching Lived Experience: Human Science for an Action Sensitive Pedagogy* (second ed.). London, Ontario, Canada: Althouse Press.

———. (Ed.). (2002) *Writing in the Dark: Phenomenological Studies in Interpretive Inquiry*. London, Ontario, Canada: Althouse Press.

III

EMPOWERMENT IN
WORKWORLDS: SELF-OTHER
TRANSFORMATIONS IN
CORPORATE ENVIRONMENTS

7

The Lifeworld of High-Performance Teams

An Experiential Account

Lucy Dinwiddie

MY QUEST TO UNDERSTAND HIGH PERFORMANCE: BEGINNING REFLECTIONS

I believe that there is a misconception about the experience of high performance within a team context, the misconception being that, when one is a member of a high-performance team, the experience is always a positive one, enhancing both the individual's life and the group's viability. Moreover, I have found that, in management literature, high-performance teams are often discussed with cult-like reverence. This view perpetuates a myth, creating a bias toward high performance and elation around its virtues, an *ideal team* fantasy (similar to the *perfect marriage* fantasy), perhaps at a dear cost of human spirit. Reflecting on my team membership history, I realized that there is a dual nature to the high-performing team experience.

Several years ago, I was part of an intense, intricate, difficult consulting project that called for constant twelve- to fourteen-hour workdays, six or even seven days a week. As my spirit and energy waned, we, as a team, were achieving the seemingly impossible goals that had been set. This paradoxical dynamic caused me to gyrate between joy and despair. As a consulting team, we were definitely delivering high-quality work against an aggressive workplan. However, I couldn't help but wonder about the cost of this high performance, to me and the others, and what drove us to accomplish these goals. Our leader pushed us hard. Our clients expected *speed to value*. Team members experienced individual and group success, but there was also conflict, hard feelings, competition, and distrust. Were we a high-performance team? If we got the job done, did it matter if we were not functioning smoothly on the human side? Which criteria—the human dynamics, the work results, or the blending of both—should be used to determine if we were a high-performance team? And who was to judge us as a high performance team? Was it our client, our leader, the consulting firm, individual team members, the team as a whole, or me?

While living through this powerful, at times painful, and highly productive team experience, all of my team experiences began to move to the foreground and haunt my mind, creating a passion and excitement that made it necessary for me to initiate and fully engage in a phenomenological inquiry (Dinwiddie, 2000).

PHENOMENOLOGY: THE RIGHT CHOICE FOR MY INQUIRY

Peter Vaill's groundbreaking exploration of high performance teams is relevant to my inquiry. In a piece entitled "Toward a Behavioral Description of High Performing Systems," Vaill sought to explicate the events or behaviors that may be observed in a system that performs well against predetermined goals. He articulated eight assumptions with deep roots in the field of organizational development. According to Vaill, these assumptions are no longer sufficient to characterize what happens when people work well and create high performance. Instead, he stressed a philosophy that advocates self-analysis and inclusion of other voices, which aligns strongly with the use of a phenomenological framework for inquiry. In Vaill's words,

> to understand a human system, and particularly a high performance human system, I think we need richer and more vivid accounts of how the system is actually operating. . . . Vivid narrative in which the writer's value system is not disguised holds out more promise, to me, for understanding a high performance system, . . . than any controlled experiment with independent and dependent variables. . . . [In high performance teams,] there obviously was a synergy operating that can only be understood by studying the situation in all of its richness and complexity. (1978, 119–24)

In light of Vaill's thought, and my own team experiences, I realized that there was an important gap in the understanding of high performance within a team, which phenomenology could help to close. Inspired by Vaill, I examined the phenomenon of high performance within a team, as described by individuals who have directly experienced it as team members. Central to my inquiry is not why the team was deemed *high performing*, but rather what occurred within an individual's lifeworld.

In its classic usage, the term *phenomenology* means the study of modes of appearing, from the Greek word *phenomenon*, meaning appearance. This movement traces its roots to Edmund Husserl (1965, 1975), who developed the phenomenological method as a means to gain knowledge of invariant structures of consciousness. This method entails placing individual consciousness, and one's perception and apprehension of world, at the center of investigation (Bentz and Shapiro, 1998). Thus, I needed to begin my inquiry by returning to myself and employing a reflective process that both elucidated my own high-performance experiences and portrayed the structures of lived experience among team members.

Instead of classifying experience according to symptoms, a descriptive or existential-phenomenological approach attends to the life structures through which experience is organized, aiming to uncover the basic structures of human existence. According to Schutz, only by comprehending the motives of an actor do we grasp the subjective meaning of the phenomenon (as cited in Polkinghorne, 1983). It was my hope that, by grounding this study in phenomenology, the subjective meaning of the individual team members' stories would be called out, examined, and understood. Sheree Dukes (1984) suggested that phenomenological methodology differs from traditional methodologies since it seeks to *see* the logical structure or meaning of an experience, rather than seeking to discover causal connections or patterns of correlation. The nature of this type of task demands extensive study of a small sample, allowing individuals to speak for themselves and to reveal the logic (or structure) of their experience *as lived*.

My work was guided by Clark Moustakas's approach to phenomenology, which is rooted in the work of Husserl. Phenomenological method requires that the researcher look beneath layers of preconceptions and assumptions to direct experience (1994, 26). Using intuition, and focusing attention to what one actually apprehends, are necessary to the discovery of knowledge (46).

MY METHOD OF INQUIRY: UNFOLDING THE PROCESS

Since the inquiry focused on discovering an individual's experience of high performance within a team context, I interviewed twenty-two team members, across a range of organizations, who believed that they had participated in a high-performance team and were willing to share their personal experiences with me in an open way. During each interview, I questioned the participants about why they believed that their experiences were of team high performance; whether others (such as team members, customers, and/or leaders) would describe the group as a *high-performance team*; and if so, why, or if not, why not. Although I was less concerned about whether people on the outside would have described the team as high performance, I found that the participants' reflections about the external world's validation of high performance was very important to everyone interviewed.

Organizational-criteria inclusion data, such as cost savings, productivity, and increased profitability, which are often used as the primary qualifiers for determining high performance, were not primary or overt selection criteria for my study. In addition, I did not use traditional personal-criteria inclusion data, such as profession, education level, socioeconomic bracket, age, gender, or race. Rather, the essential criteria for inclusion in the study were (a) a belief that one had been part of a high-performance team, (b) a willingness to engage in an initial two-hour interview process (centered on one's personal experience of high performance within a team context) and follow-up conversations as required, and (c) the ability to reflect on and articulate their high-performance experience.

It is important to note that the transactional nature of my inquiry (the two-hour, in-depth interview process) facilitated rich dialogue with participants, who co-created the interview and helped determine the directions that we explored. Creating this dialogue was essential, since human behavior and feelings, unlike physical objects, cannot be truly understood without reference to the meanings and purposes attached by the individual to her activities and experience (Guba and Lincoln, 1998). Consequently, each dialogue was dialectical in nature, transforming my current paradigms and biases into a more mindful, informed consciousness. We created and understood our realities through our discussion. As Skolimowski (1992) emphasized, our (mine and the team members') understanding and reality were products of the exchange between each of us and our collective mind. Within our discussions, there was reciprocity, such that both of us voiced and heard the other's exchange of ideas and insights, co-creating the interview dialogue, which meant that my inquiry's process was personal and intentional, and each participant's perspective was integral to our individual worldview and collective experience (Reason, 1998).

While we may be creating lifeworlds and acting out dramas within the workplace, we do so within some context. The philosopher Georg Hegel (1977) claimed that we must consider a phenomenon not in isolation, but rather within the larger social system and historical context that gives it life and meaning. Thus, it was important that I consider, as much as possible, the complete context in which team high performance occurred by attempting to understand, analyze, and critique the elements or environments that fostered an individual's positive or negative high-performance team experiences.

Since each team member's story was situated in social, economic, political, technological, and psychological structures, it was critically important to discern high-performance experience elements such as greatness, freedom, growth, joyfulness, and social justice, as well as what may have contributed to their occurrence. Likewise, it was critically important to discern high-performance experience features such as oppression, domination, exploitation, and injustice, and again what may have contributed to their occurrence.

As I carefully assessed my thoughts, searched for similarities and differences, connections and disconnections, unique and common themes, and summarized my discoveries, I found that I needed to go back and forth in my thinking. These movements—forward and backward, in and out, up and down—were fundamental to my mindfulness, allowing me to be strongly present in the study as both a team member and an inquirer (Bentz and Shapiro, 1998). By embodying mindfulness, I hoped to be in a state of care and acceptance, co-creating a time and space such that all study participants were able to shine forth and honestly reveal themselves to me in a trustful way. I believed that, by being mindful, I would be better able to move both the inquiry and us to the deep and more significant realm of human dignity and respect.

Most importantly, from my analysis of the interview data and my personal journaling and reflections, six caricatures or Schutzian *puppets* emerged that depict high-performing team member *ideal types* as well as the critical theme of *reconceptualization of self*.

THE LIFEWORLD OF A HIGH-PERFORMANCE TEAM: A SCHUTZIAN PERSPECTIVE

In 1964, Alfred Schutz described a methodology for developing ideal types by imaginatively creating puppets. Schutz's intent and process for the forming of ideal types was to "replace the human beings, which the social scientist observes as actors on the social stage" and construct the ideal types of these actors (17–19). At the highest level, the process involves observing human events and activities, and ascribing *invariable motives* to the mind of an imaginary actor, typifying a unique consciousness and predilection to action. This consciousness is "restricted in its content only to those elements necessary for the performance of the typical acts under consideration" (17–19). Thus, the puppet type exemplifies, in a microcosm, what a real person or actor would do in the real social world.

Because the forming of ideal types is central to my inquiry, I feel that it is important to explicate this conception by citing Schutz directly, in some detail:

> It is one of the outstanding features of modern social science to have described the device the social scientists use in building up their conceptual scheme, and it is the great merit of [Durkheim, Pareto, Marshall, Veblen, and] above all Max Weber, to have developed this technique in all its fullness and clarity. This technique consists in replacing the human beings, which the social scientist observes as actors on the social stage by puppets created by himself, in other words, in constructing ideal types of actors. This is done in the following way.

The scientist observes certain events within the social world as caused by human activity and he begins to establish a type of such events. Afterwards he coordinates with these typical acts typical because motives and in-order-to motives which he assumes as invariable in the mind of an imaginary actor. Thus he constructs a personal ideal type, which means the model of an actor whom he imagines as gifted with a consciousness. But it is a consciousness restricted in its content only to all those elements necessary for the performance of the typical acts under consideration. These elements it contains completely, but nothing beyond them. . . . For from the first the puppet type is imagined as having the same specific knowledge of the situation—including means and conditions—which a real actor would have in the real social world; from the first the subjective motives of a real actor performing a typical act are implanted as constant elements of the specious consciousness of the personal ideal type; . . . And as the type is constructed in such a way that it performs exclusively typical acts, the objective and subjective elements in the formation of unit-acts coincide. (1964, 17–18)

Seeking to adhere to Schutz's methodology, I reviewed each individual's transcript and identified distinct themes that were special to that person's experience and pervasive throughout the interview. However, at first I was not able to integrate these emerging themes into coherent ideal types; it was only by diligently following Schutz's description of the social scientist's creation of puppets that I was able to bring together the content of the interviews and themes such that a mosaic-like picture emerged. Each theme alone was like a singular mosaic tile but, when added together, they created six ideal types, revealing a complex picture of lifeworlds with perspective and depth. Each of the puppets incorporated personal human characteristics of the team members interviewed, addressed motivations, and identified unique consciousnesses that typified them. In fact, wherever possible, actual words or phrases from an interview transcript were used to give form and voice to the constructed puppets. The six puppets, named to capture the essence of each, and their essential characteristics were

- Miss Gude Frends: relationship, bonding, connection, and community;
- Mrs. Create Legacy: lasting significance, innovation, difference, and destiny;
- Professor Free Domm: autonomy, professional discretion, growth, and space;
- Mr. Gotta Trackit: project management, schedules, timelines, and relentless focus on outcomes;
- Mr. Deep Meaning: joyfulness, spiritual link, and connection to life and purpose; and

- Mrs. Must Winn: importance of success, being the best, and controlling to ensure victory.

For illustrative purposes, I display four of the six puppets below, and offer summative protocols that amalgamate elements from many of my study participants to generate a single, coherent expression of the type.

Professor Free Domm

I am a competent professional who can be a strong individual performer and a strong team player. I have the ability to work tirelessly within a team to achieve individual and collective high performance as long as I am not micromanaged and controlled. I achieve my best work when a goal is communicated, limitations are outlined, and then management disengages so that the team and I can do our work. You see, the other team members and I work best when we are able to select our roles and work tasks. In addition, when the situation warrants, we must have permission to modify an individual's roles and tasks at a moment's notice. In fact, limitations imposed on this mobility and flexibility would both disappoint and stress us; such strong restrictions would severely impact my and other team members' ability (and thus the team's ability as a whole) to operate in a high-performance manner. Finally, I believe that space and autonomy, balanced with strong interpersonal and relational ties, must be based on mutual support and open communication. When this type of teaming dynamic happens, there is a blurring of roles within the team that fosters the flexibility to change and adapt, which is necessary for optimum teamwork and high performance to occur.

Mr. Gotta Trackit

I must advocate that the common language and process derived from strictly executing the project management process will provide a common basis for the team. By using project management, the work will come together and the team will produce excellent results in accordance with predetermined milestones. Project management will force intransigent and parochial team members to begin to compromise to achieve the project's quality level and fulfill the team's common purpose as documented by the workplan and Gantt charts. With strong project management, leadership will evolve to the level necessary to assure the process's execution. I think that strong interpersonal ties, which some people would espouse as crucial to high performance, are not usually the glue that connects the needed performance together. In fact, I am not sure that strong interpersonal ties are even necessary to achieve team success and high performance. I believe that even dysfunctional groups, which may be painful to members, if they employ robust project management, would still be able to produce high-quality outcomes because of the discipline imposed by the tracking mechanisms and penalties for nonconformance.

Mr. Deep Meaning

For me, personal, spiritual, and work lives are so completely interrelated as to be indistinguishable from one other. Joy, deep satisfaction, and continuous achievement flow from the resulting unity and synergy of mind, spirit, and body. Work, life, and meaning are interconnected and related. There is a sense of joy and peace in doing what I am doing: a kind of Zen, everything fitting together, all aspects of my life coming together to make the team and the work fulfilling. While my work may have a substantial transactional dimension, the important and most satisfying aspects are connections to personal calling and the interpersonal relationships that result from people collectively doing the work that they are put on earth to do. The building of, living in, and working with a community develop the common and strongly held beliefs that enable the high-performance team to define clear goals and processes. These co-created elements foster among the team members a set of shared values that are foundational to the achievement of outstanding results, while supporting a work life that is joyful and deeply satisfying. The work itself may be grand or vitally important, but it does not have to be for me to be deeply satisfied and fulfilled. The work must have, however, as a key part of its nature, the aspect of helping and/or drawing people together. I believe that using my gifts, talents, and skills, even in the simplest way, for the benefit of even just one person, is crucial to my calling. When this happens, growing personally and together as a team is not something that is done for my ego or myself. Instead, it is done as a gift to the person, the team, and/or the system that I am helping.

Mrs. Must Winn

I am driven, first, foremost, and forever, to achieve and excel. Winning and being first are crucial to my Type-A personality. I only want to be on teams that can be medal winners. I hold intense pride of ownership in the outcome of the team: Therefore, I drive myself and the team to reach high levels of performance and achievement. On the positive side, this leads the team and me to great personal and professional growth and success. On the negative side, the "I'll succeed if it kills me" attitude, coupled with a strongly felt sense of obligation to persevere, more often than not lead to burnout, personal crisis, or health issues. Over time, I am learning (if only out of necessity) that I and/or the team cannot do it all ourselves. I am beginning to learn to delegate authority to other individuals or staff. The delegation process has forced me to learn to deal with the anxiety that my letting go creates. At times, I have worked with people who do not share the same skill, knowledge, or passion for the work. This is always incredibly frustrating to me, because they do not produce the quality, quantity, or style of output that I would produce, but I am learning, at least a little, to manage the disappointment and move myself and the team forward despite the weaker team members. The teams that I am part of will always get the job done on time and within budget.

Although the puppets were created from the study's data, I must acknowledge that they also reflect something of my understanding and experience within-high performance teams. I am sure that some of the puppets' voices are projections of what I know and value; I am equally certain that some of the puppets' voices are projections of what I have rejected and cast into the shadows. I wrote the following entry in my research journal immediately after I completed puppet creation.

> I loved creating these puppets. And, I know each is a piece of me, a projection of my lifeworld on others. Despite the fact that many of the words and themes are documented in the interview transcripts verbatim, I co-created the interviews and decided what elements were important to call out.
>
> I know I need professional freedom: to micromanage me is to imprison my creativity and spirit. Much of my energy goes into escape (mentally or physically) and not results. I need to be liked. My teams need to have a spirit of camaraderie. I want to like and enjoy the people around me. This friendship does help me take risks, grow, develop.
>
> Project management: a double-edged sword for me. It does provide common vision and grounding for the work and decision-making, and it can be a vise that grips the team's heart tightly. I could never be Mr. Gotta Trackit, but my organizations want me to be him.
>
> I believe to the bottom of my soul that I am doing the work I was put on earth to do. Organization development is my vocation and avocation. I believe I was meant to do this study. I believe it is part of my calling.
>
> I do want to make a difference. I have learned that I can't change the world, my company, my church, but I can change my part of the organization, the teams I lead, the groups I support.
>
> Do I need to win? Is this yet another shadow part of me as the project management puppet? I want high evaluations on my performance reviews and to advance. I will have four degrees including a PhD. I continue to challenge myself on many fronts. So yes, this too is part of me. (Excerpts from personal research journal)

The purpose of constructing Schutzian sociological ideal types is to bridge individual-specific constructs of actors with more common, generic constructs that are robust enough to reflect and exemplify the experience of multiple actors who experience a similar context or situation. The four constructed types draw from my own experiences on high-performance teams and those of my study participants. In addition, by applying the Schutzian puppets to the accounts given by my study participants, I discovered several overarching themes in the data. The most central was the idea of reconceptualizing the self.

WHAT MAKES HIGH-PERFORMING TEAM MEMBERS: RECONCEPTUALIZATION OF SELF

For me, the most powerful single theme that I encountered surfaced as I interviewed Sam, who stated that he believed that, during his high-performance team experience, he was able to reconceptualize his image of himself. Sam said that he found pieces of himself that he had lost, and discovered talents and skills that he did not even know he had. Sam recalled that, because of the team's input, mentoring, support, and concern for him, he was able to redefine "who Sam is, and what Sam is capable of doing."

Because of the depth of Sam's belief that he grew, developed, and changed during his high-performance team experience, I consciously began to explore whether other individuals had experienced this dynamic. Often, a participant vividly described the idea that her view of herself had changed while being part of a high-performance team experience. The participant's positive reconceptualization of self (the adding of skills, knowledge, talents, risk tolerance, and so forth), and the associated enhancement of self-esteem, resulted in an increased ability to contribute to the team's vision and goals. Sam said that he believed it was this positive reconceptualization of self that was the "magic pixie dust" that created synergy, which is often defined as "the whole being greater than the sum of the parts." Sam said that although he understood the concept of synergy, he had always wondered where the extra portion came from. From his high-performance experience, Sam shared that he now knows that the extra portion surfaces during team experiences and feels that he is more than the sum of his original parts.

In addition, the positive reconceptualization of self seems to affect not just the work part of the individual, but rather it enables the whole self (work, spiritual, intellectual, and emotional) to evolve and grow with team members' feedback and support. Many team members said that this was an important feature of their high-performance experience within a team context, as these excerpts illustrate:

Carol: I was totally overwhelmed, totally overwhelmed, because I was challenged to do things that I had never, even in my wildest dreams, thought that, in my lifetime, that I would be able to do. Yet, I was able to find something in myself, or others saw something in me, that I never knew I had or that I could do something with.

Drew: I think I changed, as well. . . . I became far less directed and far more visionary—kind of empowering people, letting them do their job, and staying out of the way. It was amazing, just how much each person could do as they grew, developed, and became stronger professionals. As a matter of fact, I changed and grew as well.

Sally: He was completely trusting; he said, "You and I know it will be good." And he helped me see it as an opportunity. What he did was change the lens through which I was looking at this experience, so that I was able to maximize it for the engagement, for the client, and for me, instead of looking at it as something negative. That was a gift. That was really a gift. I learned that I am more than I think that I am. I can do more than I think I can. I can give more than I think I can give.

In like fashion, when a participant had been part of negative team situations, the reconceptualization had also been present. Instead of being a growth experience (wherein parts of oneself are found and added to the self-concept), the experience is one of lessening or minimizing the image of self, with detrimental consequences to the individual. As I explored this negative reconceptualization of self, it seemed that those experiencing it continued to work hard, contribute, and meet deadlines and deliverables according to schedule, but completed the tasks without the discovery of new talents, skills, or competencies. The high-performance results came from long, hard, grueling hours and high personal sacrifice, not from the added dimensions of an enhanced and/or revitalized sense of self. Several excerpts illustrate the many individual experiences of a diminished self-conception:

Amy: I took on a lot of hurt because, you'd ask people to do things, and they'd tell you that you were stupid or wrong or inexperienced or you didn't know what you were doing, but you did. My self-image during this time was at an all-time low. It took me years to regain some parts of it. The situation was so painful to me that, even fifteen years later, I have never set foot in that place. It would just remind me of a low point in my life.

Jay: I always like to think I have some ability to influence or control it or to make it occur. But, I'll tell you, in that situation, the odd thing for me was that I felt like I had all the competencies to do it, but nothing I could do seemed to help. If anything, everything I tried to do to help it seemed to hurt it, because in doing that very thing, it seemed to open up yet some other issues. It sort of seemed like we were in a death spiral.

James: People became very, very frustrated with attempting to get issues resolved or approved. We had an entire hierarchy through which issues had to be
worked, and it was very frustrating at times, causing people to check out temporarily. And when deadlines weren't met or the project wasn't meeting expectations, our lives were made very miserable by management. People began to
get stressed out and blame each other, but we did work twice as hard and man-
aged to get it done, if just to stop the pain.

DISPELLING THE MYTH OF HIGH-PERFORMANCE ELATION: FEAR AND PAIN EXPOSED

Within my own experience of high-performance teams, I have lived through
both negative and positive team scenarios. In the course of conducting
twenty-two in-depth interviews, thirty-eight team experiences were discussed; in quantitative terms, twenty-six (or 68 percent) were described as
positive, and twelve (or 32 percent) negative.

To revisit and describe the negative team experiences, an individual must
go back to a painful place, relive it, and wonder if she will be believed or
held to blame for the negative dynamics. Many of the participants, both
male and female, related negative team experiences in a very emotional way.
Some stated that fear was a contributing factor; in such interviews, fear was
an omnipresent element in the transcribed text. Several times, as participants discussed the power of their fear, I got chills up and down my spine
as I was drawn into their emotions and their pain. When I reviewed the interview transcripts, the multiple sources of fear emerged. Participants most
often cited a fear of (a) being embarrassed or humiliated (in public or in
private); (b) not achieving what was promised, or letting someone down;
(c) saying or doing something unpopular and suffering the resulting reper-
cussions for voicing or doing it; and (d) loss of status, advancement, or
livelihood/job.

Surprisingly, when fear was present, the team member still continued to
perform and achieve, but at great expense to his personal state. Added to the
overpowering need to achieve was the astonishing willingness to sacrifice
one's self in the face of clearly unreasonable expectations. During the interviews, participants told stories of negative (mental or physical) health consequences, broken relationships, lack of personal time and space, change of
job or career, development of prejudices, and reluctance to take risks. Nevertheless, all individuals performed as directed. Their fear was closely associated with unhealthy and exploitative situations wherein they felt at great
risk to do anything other than accept the status quo.

Fear also prevented open and honorable conversations, which might
have led to change. The following quotes illustrate the power of fear:

Kelly: It got so uncomfortable for Beej, being part of this team and this process, which he couldn't really support or defend, that his back literally twisted up. He actually became deformed, like the Hunchback of Notre Dame. He was in severe pain because he was not able to let go of his fears about the project being successful. He just didn't see how this was going to work. And that stress and fear manifested itself in harming his health.

Ann: Big-time fear of failure. I'm a perfectionist. I was scared for myself that, in order to make the things happen that needed to, I would put my needs and the needs of my family to the side. I knew myself well enough to know that, to be successful, I might sacrifice my family and myself, which ultimately did happen. Also, everything suffered, including my health and mental well-being. . . . I felt like I was between a rock and a hard place. I just put myself on work autopilot and just went forward. . . . But what resulted is that I was so focused on success that our marriage crashed on the rocks.

Beth: Everything was demanded. Fear ruled, mandating higher quality and improvement. . . . Everything was just geared that way. You don't just do your job; you must do it much better than your job, or you get a "meets standards" review, which, to me, is just unacceptable when you are working your tail off. If I get a "meets standards," I feel terrible, like I'm not doing my job well, and how can that be when I work hours and hours and hours? And we all know that, with such reviews, you don't get promoted. I guess that I just have to exceed the impossible standards that are set, or I will be extremely disappointed in myself and deemed a failure by others.

Fear, in its manifest forms, surfaced as a key ingredient in reports of negative team-based experiences and the minimization aspects of reconceptualization of self. Fear also served as a catalyst for my own understanding and learnings from my research, as I sought to be consciously part of high-performing teams that are not detrimental to me and others. In closing, I turn to some of the more salient phenomenological outcomes that are serving as an impetus to my own personal change and that of lifeworlds that intersect with or are impacted by mine.

PHENOMENOLOGICAL OUTCOMES: LEARNING ABOUT OTHERS AND CHANGING MYSELF

One of the most important aspects of an inquiry is the responsibility and ethics of the inquirer. Throughout my study, I have been at the center of the process. My awareness of self (personal, social, intellectual, emotional, and historical) has shaped my inquiry and research in powerful ways. Likewise, my study of scholarly traditions such as phenomenology has shaped the inquiry in profound ways. During the study, I learned about the essence of the

individual's experience of high performance within a team context by talking to individuals who have been part of such experiences, discerning patterns and themes, and relating them back to the literature.

In addition, I wanted to understand what makes the high-performance
experience positive or negative for the individual. I believed that, by whole-
heartedly engaging myself in the study, the business and social science communities could more readily understand the myth, mystery, and mandates
of high-performance groups. I wondered if new insights into what constitutes an individual's experience of a healthy and functional high-
performance group could be extrapolated to an organizational experience
of high achievement. And I wondered whether or not I could harness new
insights to do such an extrapolation. The hope was that I could conduct an
inquiry that would explore the conception of high performance or high
achievement in a more open and thoughtful way.

As a result of my research, I have come to believe fervently that the
shadow side of high performance must be more fully explored and discussed. The idea that business is about people has been around for a long
time, and yet rarely are people adequately considered in strategic business
decisions. With social forces like globalization, the new economy, and the
information society, is it any wonder that the organization and its work-
force feel increasingly insecure and threatened? Added to these dynamics is
the continuing, relentless power of the mechanistic model of business that
encourages managers to see people as machines that are interchangeable
and replaceable. Thus, it is easy for an organization and its management
team to focus exclusively on the producing of goods or services and forget
that a team is a community of human beings. Is it any wonder that, out of
the thirty-eight team experiences discussed by my study participants, 32
percent were negative? Imagine spending one third of your work life
doomed to negative team experiences. When would you choose to opt out?

The fear and pain that my participants related to me was real, powerful,
and appalling. What organizational or team accomplishment could be
worth that cost? The loss of health, marriage, and family is a terrible toll for
success. The loss of pride in oneself, minimization of one's identity, and
fearfulness to reach out or try new things constitute a waste of human potential. The accounts of my study participants are etched in my heart and
mind. Their voices fuel the need to study and examine the shadow side of
high-performance work teams, which will surely be emancipating as the
stock of knowledge develops.

I believe that my team experience over the past two years illustrates the
integrity of the exploration, reflections, and findings that I have advanced.
Alfred Schutz, who brought the philosophy of phenomenology into the social science arena, explained this connection:

If I look at my whole stock of your lived experiences and ask about the structure of this knowledge, one thing becomes clear: This is that everything I know about your conscious life is really based on my knowledge of my own lived experiences. My lived experiences of you are constituted in simultaneity or quasi-simultaneity with your lived experiences, to which they are intentionally related. It is only because of this that, when I look backward, I am able to synchronize my experiences of you with your experiences. (1967, 106)

Thus, by conducting a phenomenological study and learning deeply about the human experience of high performance, my team experience and the experience of others on our team become more consciously lived, with stronger, healthier, and more robust results.

REFERENCES

Bentz, Valerie M., and Jeremy J. Shapiro. (1998) *Mindful Inquiry in Social Research.* Thousand Oaks, CA: Sage.

Dinwiddie, Lucille. (2000) *A Mindful Inquiry into Understanding How the Individual Constructs the Experience of High Performance Within a Team Context.* Unpublished Ph.D. Dissertation. Santa Barbara, CA: The Fielding Institute.

Dukes, Sheree. (1984) Phenomenological Methodology in the Human Sciences. *Journal of Religion and Health, 23*(3), 197–203.

Guba, Egon G., and Yvonna S. Lincoln. (1998) Competing Paradigms in Qualitative Research. In N. K. Denzin and Y. S. Lincoln (Eds.), *The Landscape of Qualitative Research: Theories and Issues.* Thousand Oaks, CA: Sage.

Hegel, Georg W. F. (1977) Who Thinks Abstractly? In W. Kaufmann (Trans. and Ed.), *Hegel: Texts and Commentary.* Chicago: University of Notre Dame Press.

Husserl, Edmund. (1965) *Phenomenology and the Crisis of Philosophy.* New York: Harper & Row.

———. (1975) *The Paris Lectures.* The Hague, The Netherlands: Martinus Hijhoff.

Moustakas, Clark. (1994) *Phenomenological Research Methods.* Thousand Oaks, CA: Sage.

Polkinghorne, Donald. (1983) *Methodology for the Human Sciences: Systems of Inquiry.* Albany: State University of New York Press.

Reason, Peter. (1998) Three Approaches to Participative Inquiry. In N. K. Denzin and Y. S. Lincoln (Eds.), *Strategies of Qualitative Inquiry.* Thousand Oaks, CA: Sage.

Schutz, Alfred. (1964) *Collected Papers II: Studies in Social Theory.* The Hague, The Netherlands: Martinus Nijhoff.

———. (1967) *A Phenomenology of the Social World.* (G. Walsh and F. Lehnert, Trans.) Evanston, IL: Northwestern University Press.

Skolimowski, H. (1992) *Living Philosophy: Eco-Philosophy as a Tree of Life.* London: Arkana.

Vaill, Peter B. (1978) Toward a Behavioral Description of High-Performance Systems. In M. McCall and M. Lombardo (Eds.), *Leadership: Where Else Can We Go?* Durham, NC: Duke University Press.

8

Personal Power

Realizing Self in Doing and Being

Bernie Novokowsky

> Everybody seems to know what it [power] is except the experts. They debate definitions endlessly, and how it differs from influence, control, authority, etc. Yet ordinary people seem to have no trouble with the concept. They know what it means to have power.
>
> Henry Mintzberg (1983)

I was an exception to Mintzberg's claim. As an ordinary person, I did not understand what it means "to have power," but my study of phenomenology and hermeneutics changed all that. My interest in studying the topic of personal power arose from dissatisfaction with some of my life experiences. Upon reflection, I came to see two recurring themes throughout my life: my actions have not achieved the desired result on many occasions, and I lacked a clear and adequate sense of *being*. As such, I have often felt lacking in personal power, something that I became very aware of when I was eight or nine years old. I offer the following account of a childhood event that has shaped my life, and why researching the topic of personal power became a necessity later in my life.

> I recall what happened one warm, typical summer evening. My father had just come home from the beer parlor about 8:00 p.m. He was extremely angry about something, and started yelling loudly at my mother, but mostly at us kids. I was confused. We had done nothing wrong, so I did not understand why he was so angry with us. Then he started hitting and kicking my mother, really beating her up. I was really scared of his violence. Soon, the police had arrived. Then a Catholic priest drove up. This priest knew our family well, especially my

mother. I remember watching the police and priest talking to my parents, trying to calm my father down. They were also talking to a couple of the neigh-
bors and my brothers and sisters. It seemed like a real zoo to me.

When the police and priest first arrived, I was glad. I felt they would take care
of things and ensure my mother and all of us were safe. As things calmed
down, the priest came over and asked me what had happened. I explained how
my father had come home and, for no apparent reason, starting beating up my
mom. The priest told me that my mother must have done something to cause
this incident, because my father was a good man. I could not do anything to
change his view that my father was innocent and my mother was the villain.
The police left shortly thereafter, saying they could not do anything. Later, I
learned my mother was too afraid to press any charges.

I remember feeling angry and hurt that no punishment had been given to
my father for his violence, and how both the priest and police seemed to support my father rather than my mother. I knew it was wrong. I wanted to correct
the injustice, yet felt totally powerless to do anything. I wasn't big enough to
fight my father back. I couldn't run away, as I didn't feel I could take care of
myself, nor would that help my mother. As well, I felt betrayed by both the
priest and police, who were supposed to be right and good. In short, I felt help-
less, hurt, and powerless. There was nothing I could do.

As an adult, my frustration with my sense of a lack of personal power has
continued. In this essay, I share my search to understand my situation, and
how learning and applying phenomenological and hermeneutic strategies
resulted in a completed doctoral research dissertation (Novokowsky, 1999),
one that has helped me resolve many of these lifelong, lingering issues. My
hope is that, by sharing my discoveries, others can understand how certain
styles of research can be harnessed to more deeply grasp one's ordinary and
eventful life experiences.

WRITING PHENOMENOLOGICAL PROTOCOLS: EXPLORATIONS OF PERSONAL POWER

Personal power is central to our daily lives, affecting productivity, mood,
sense of well-being, and relations to others. Our initial sense of and experience with personal power are derived from our lifeworld experiences, especially what we learn from others. We are enveloped by the consequences of
having, and not having, sufficient personal power to manage our daily affairs. As the opening account of my childhood experience with family violence displays, I experienced, but did not understand, what was happening
to me. Understanding the meaning of experience requires a special reflective effort, something that phenomenological and hermeneutic inquiry can
provide.

The methodology of my study is located within the qualitative research tradition of *hermeneutic phenomenology* (Bentz and Shapiro, 1998; van Manen, 1990). My quest to understand the meaning of *personal power* also led me to explore research on evolutionary development and hierarchy theory (Ahl and Allen, 1996; Simon, 1973). Figure 8.1 provides an overview of the elements that entered into my study (scheme adopted from Bennett, 1993, 1997).

I began my research by taking stock of my own life experiences, and isolating peak experiences where a sense of powerlessness or power was evident. Building upon twelve such experiences, I then developed what are called *phenomenological protocols* (van Manen, 1990, 64–65). The purpose of protocol writing is to generate original text on which the researcher can then work. *Protocols* are rich, thick descriptions of personal experience, which capture one's own view of experience as lived from the inside. These are direct accounts, using active voice, which speak from the viewpoint of "I." Each of my protocols was rewritten a number of times to clarify parts, to amplify parts, and add new parts. I *bracketed* aspects of the experience to clarify the essential structure of personal power (Bentz, 1989; Husserl, 1970).

After I completed writing my personal protocols, the next step was to do a hermeneutic analysis of each protocol. I followed the directives in Hans-Georg Gadamer's analysis, specifically what he called *Three Levels of the I-Thou* (1975). Table 8.1 displays the three levels. I focused on level 3, taking the *listener role*, as I worked with each of my protocols.

Three protocols from different phases of my life are offered here to display what descriptive protocol writing entails. Protocol 1 is a recollection of

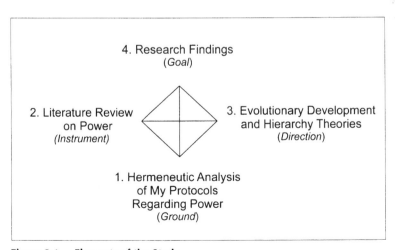

Figure 8.1. Elements of the Study

Table 8.1.   Gadamer's Three Levels of the I-Thou

	"I" Researcher (Myself)	Relation	"THOU" The Text (My Protocols)
Level 1	Observer role	→→→→→→→→→→ Descriptive Objectivity	My objective lived- experience descriptions
Level 2	Reflector role	→→→→→→→→→→ Dialectic Reflection ◄┄◄┄◄┄◄┄◄┄◄┄◄┄◄┄◄┄	My reflections: patterns and themes
Level 3	Listener role	→→→→→→→→→→ Authentic Opening ⇦⇦⇦⇦⇦⇦⇦⇦⇦	My hermeneutic experience

camping experiences with friends during my youth. Protocol 2 addresses experience within my activity as a professional external consultant. Protocol
3 speaks to my experience and practice with traditional Chinese qi gong. At
the end of each protocol, I display a sampling of what the hermeneutic
analysis revealed from my examination of my self-generated texts.

Protocol 1: Camping Overnight

I grew up on the northern edge of our city, a few blocks from the river. As kids,
my friends and I would go north along the riverbanks and explore. The farther
we went from the city, the more I felt like an adventurer. Also, the farther we
went, the more I felt at risk and vulnerable because it was a long way back to
get help. Regardless, we would go on exploring and playing. When I was about
ten years old, I went on my first overnight camping trip along the river. I had
camped with adults, but this was the first time camping with only a friend my
age.

My friend and I walked up the river for several hours, farther up river than
either of us had ever been before. We found and established a campsite, built
a fire, and cooked supper. Then we gathered more wood, improved our campsite, and did some line fishing. However, the blackness of night soon came. We
sat around the fire and talked, while keeping it burning brightly. I recall how
the fire provided me warmth and comfort. It also illuminated our immediate
surroundings extremely well.

Eventually it was time to sleep. My friend and I got into our sleeping bags. It
was only then that I really noticed the sounds in the wooded thickets around
us. The fire began to burn down. The air got colder and the surroundings got
blacker. Suddenly, there was a particularly loud rustling in the thickets. We
didn't know what it was, but it sounded like it was caused by something big.
My friend said he was frightened. I was too.

I felt scared, not knowing what was out there, and knew I could not rely on
my frightened friend to take care of me. So I realized that I had to deal with it.

I do not recall when I stopped being scared, but I do remember thinking that it was only sounds, and that there was nothing in our sight that proved we were in any real danger. Somehow, I both knew, and felt, that I had to be strong. I reassured my friend that everything was fine, and that if something came at us we had our small axe and knives to defend ourselves. By saying this out loud, I felt stronger. Nonetheless, I stood on guard for a time. I kept thinking about the possibilities and what we could do in the eventuality of each possibility. I worked at keeping myself calm. After a while, the noises and night chills passed from my attention and I went to sleep. In the morning, I felt really alive and powerful. I had "survived" the first night out on my own and had overcome the fears. I felt I was able to take care of myself.

Hermeneutic Analysis of Protocol 1

In performing level 3 Gadamerian analyses on this protocol, I first looked for key words or phrases that said something about my experience of power. Then, I looked at patterns that emerged from these highlighted words or phrases. From these patterned clusters, key points were identified. Throughout these three steps, I made a conscious effort to *bracket*—to set aside—what I thought I knew about power and look at what my protocols were really telling me. What I discovered from this analysis was that, as I accepted my fear and vulnerability, power emerged when I took the risk to act. I could empower myself by taking action in the face of danger. A stronger, though still vulnerable, self arose from this action.

There is a notable difference between feeling powerless against my father's rage and the first protocol of overcoming fear while camping. Although I was a child in both, the camping experience of power entailed making choices and, thus, seeing viable options. When I experienced powerlessness, I had no choices. The key thing that differentiated my experience of power and powerlessness was my own assessment of the situation, and not necessarily the situation itself.

Protocol 2: Executive Coaching

During my first three years as a full-time, external management consultant, I offered a wide variety of services. In three subsequent years, I focused on business redesign and implementation. During this six-year period, coaching managers had only been a secondary service—means to other ends. Later, I received a call from a human resources department, asking if I would be interested in doing an executive coaching assignment. The process was to recommend three different consultants to the executive. Their plan was to have all three individuals interviewed by the executive, who would then select the person who would serve as coach.

The executive officer was a high-profile person in a large, profit-generating institution. He was in his mid-forties and had a reputation for being highly

Bernie Novokowsky

intelligent and energetic. He was a recognized expert within his field, and on the board of directors for about fifteen organizations. This person was well known and accomplished. However, both he and his superiors recognized that he needed some further development. Over an extended lunch, we met with the intent of interviewing each other. During our conversation, he told me that he was looking for some meaningful help, and not in the form of giving him tools, techniques, or models to follow. He went on to say he was intellectually aware of his shortfalls, but was not being authentic in addressing them. I felt tense and my anxiety rose when he said this. I had built my consulting practice on one-page answers for a multitude of problems and issues. Nothing in this arsenal of quick answers could address what I had just been told.

Listening to him speak about the details of his issues, I realized that my files, that have served me so well in the past, would be of little value to me should I get this contract. The thought frightened me. It challenged me to wonder: "Who am I, as a consultant, without my portfolio of one-pagers? What value am I as a person, compared to the value of my tools and techniques?" These questions were racing around in the back of my mind while we were conversing.

During our dialogue, I sensed that he really was highly intelligent. This triggered inner feelings of insecurity and fueled more interior dialogue while I was talking with him. My inner dialogue was questioning, "Who am I to think I can help someone who is far more accomplished than I am? In performing this contract, there will only be the bare me as the source of help—what if I am not good enough?" Yet, among these strong voices of doubt and fear, another voice surfaced: "I am all that I have to work with, and that 'who I am' is good." The voice reminded me that I had done a lot of reflection and work on improving myself over the years, and that I did not have to hide behind my methods, tools, and techniques. All I needed to do was to be present and authentic. The strong voices of doubt and fear responded, and this inner debate continued, all the while I was in conversation with this executive.

My lunch conversation with this executive continued. I asked him questions and took notes. When he questioned me, I found myself not being able to answer in my usual consulting role. Rather, I was answering from "who I am." While monitoring my inner dialogue, I decided to test "who I am" to see if it was a good fit. The underlying issue was about authenticity, and not consulting fees and interventions.

At the end of our two-hour meeting, he announced that he was very comfortable with me, and that he wanted to proceed with contracting me to be his coach. He said he did not have to interview the other two consultants. He requested I use my notes and draft a short coaching contract for us to review in a week's time. When I left that meeting, I still had some feelings of anxiety about being good enough to perform this contract. Yet I had a great sense of presence—strong feelings that just "being me" was good enough for today—and if it was good enough for today, then, with work, I could make it good enough for my next coaching meeting.

Hermeneutic Analysis of Protocol 2

From my analysis of this protocol, I gleaned the insight that my experience of power came from trusting my real self, as opposed to relying on the opinions of others. Fear, doubt, and insecurity are integral to the experience. There is a tension between two competing voices in my inner dialogue. One voice advocates playing it safe and sticking with what I am comfortable with doing. Another voice advocates exposure of my real self, which has perceived risk and the possibility of failure.

Protocol 3: Qi Gong

Qi gong is a traditional Chinese practice, with many variants, for maintaining health and fitness. My practice focuses on breathing, mental concentration, and the movement of my body's energy. When doing it, I have a greater sense of being. I find myself more relaxed, accepting, centered, and more peaceful about my world. I have a greater sense of power about my ability to deal with the world.

I try to practice qi gong for thirty minutes each day. To start, I get into the proper sitting position as prescribed by my teacher. I close my eyes and do three practice breaths and begin concentrating on focusing my energy. I begin the routine of a particular breathing type while imagining my energy slowly moving along a circular route in my body. At the same time, I try to maintain a large "inner smile" while holding a slight smile on my face. I try to get rid of all thought that is not related to my qi gong practice. Despite my concentration and focus, there are times when I catch myself slipping into thoughts about some other issue or problem. Once aware of this lapse, I refocus myself and continue.

When I finish, I feel highly energized. It is not like being at a pep rally, listening to a motivational speaker, or being caught up in the moment. It is a feeling of being highly charged, but in a very calm and sustained way. I have greater capability of taking on problematic situations. I feel that I can absorb more stress without being thrown into some irrational reaction. Having a greater sense of being, I feel a power within that I never experienced before doing qi gong.

Hermeneutic Analysis of Protocol 3

I concluded from the analysis of this protocol that my sense of power is a phenomenon that resides within me. Qi gong is a practice for my accessing and cultivating it. My notions of my *being* and *beingness* are important concepts to understanding my power. My state of being affects my state of doing, and vice versa. Reflecting on this protocol, I realized that I never would have been capable of doing or even writing about qi gong during my military career. I had only one interpretation—of being a *warrior*—and would have dismissed breathing and meditative work as nonsense. Such a view had effectively limited the scope of what personal power meant to me.

TRYING TO DO HERMENEUTICS: UNANTICIPATED INSIGHTS

From the moment that I decided to do hermeneutics, I felt uneasy, even troubled, by how I would know when I was really *doing it*. How could I go about letting my protocols just speak to me? The more I tried to design and make it happen, the more I found myself doing Gadamer's level 2 analysis, taking on the *reflector* role rather than the *listener* role outlined in level 3 (see Table 8.1). I worried about it, and wondered if I would ever complete the analysis and my doctoral research program. I decided to step away from this activity and attend to other things in my life. Then, something happened.

I was in Boston visiting with colleague, James Webber. We spent the day together, talking about my progress since my last visit. I spoke about the progress of my dissertation research and my conceptual development. James was energizing, and he stimulated my thinking. As I settled into my room later that night, I found it difficult to fall asleep. I felt compelled to get up and make notes about my experiences with power. The theme that emerged was that *I was undeveloped at the core of myself*. To become stronger, I had to allow the core of myself to be more vulnerable. It seemed paradoxical that more power and strength could be gained from allowing greater vulnerability of my *core self*. Figure 8.2 shows the conceptual sketch I made that night.

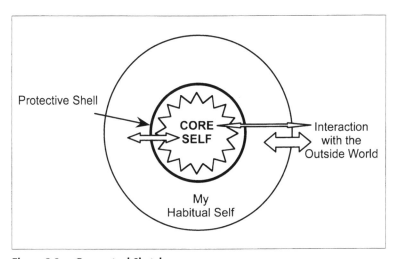

Figure 8.2.   Conceptual Sketch

The insight as to the relations between my *core self* and *habitual self* provided the breakthrough that I needed to see the connections among the elements in all twelve of the protocols generated and analyzed in my Ph.D. dissertation (Novokowsky, 1999).

Mapping Protocol Discoveries to Published Research

I chose not to review relevant research on power and personal power until after I had completed my protocol analysis. My examination of the published literature on the subject material turned out to be a broad and extensive search. I found a significant gap between my emerging understanding of power and mainstream research explanations of power. The challenge, then, became how to map the analysis of my experiential protocols to the varying definitions, concepts, and categories present in a large and complex body of formal research work. Here, I will show only one illustrative connection to reveal how knowledge from other sources served to contextualize and further extend my personal understanding. When I discovered the thought of John Bennett (1994, 1997), I sensed a way to bridge the insights of my phenomenological analysis to key insights from significant theorists on power. Bennett's work with definitional hierarchies relates, with amazing congruency, to my own hermeneutic-phenomenological analysis of power.

Drawing upon his study of systematics and ancient knowledge, Bennett asserted that there are three *hierarchical worlds*, or orderings of dimensions of human nature. In the *world of function*, there is man as machine, an instrument composed of many different subordinate instruments. This is the man we can know and study. In the *world of will*, man is will or "I," and he has possibility of being master of his instruments. In the *world of being*, man can become "being in his own right." Being allows us to complete the whole (1994, 21). These three dimensions of human nature are shown in figure 8.3.

At the simplest level, the originating etymological core of the word power is *to be able*. This etymological core can be superimposed on Bennett's three dimensions of human nature. The *to* of the *to be able* corresponds to the *will* of people and expresses what is aimed at, or intentionality. The *be* corresponds to the *being* or *beingness* of people, in a sense, the phenomenological. The *able* corresponds to the *functionality* of people, and expresses the manifestation of the will into empirical existence through us as human beings—the mechanistic paradigm. Thus, my conclusion is that this core definition of power, *to be able*, is parsimonious, a criterion that is espoused and highly regarded in hierarchy theory.

My findings uncovered the absence, or at least the understating, of *being* in the literature on power. This finding helped to explain why there was a

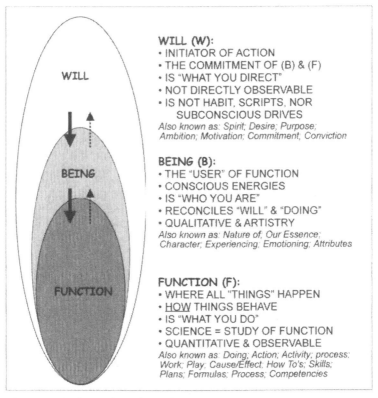

WILL (W):
• INITIATOR OF ACTION
• THE COMMITMENT OF (B) & (F)
• IS "WHAT YOU DIRECT"
• NOT DIRECTLY OBSERVABLE
• IS NOT HABIT, SCRIPTS, NOR
  SUBCONSCIOUS DRIVES
Also known as: Spirit; Desire; Purpose;
Ambition; Motivation; Commitment; Conviction

BEING (B):
• THE "USER" OF FUNCTION
• CONSCIOUS ENERGIES
• IS "WHO YOU ARE"
• RECONCILES "WILL" & "DOING"
• QUALITATIVE & ARTISTRY
Also known as: Nature of; Our Essence;
Character; Experiencing; Emotioning; Attributes

FUNCTION (F):
• WHERE ALL "THINGS" HAPPEN
• HOW THINGS BEHAVE
• IS "WHAT YOU DO"
• SCIENCE = STUDY OF FUNCTION
• QUANTITATIVE & OBSERVABLE
Also known as: Doing; Action; Activity; process;
Work; Play; Cause/Effect; How To's; Skills;
Plans; Formulas; Process; Competencies

Figure 8.3.   Three Dimensions of Human Nature

gap in my experience, which centered more on my being, and the literature, which gives nearly exclusive attention to either the functional or spirit levels of power. By adding the third dimension of being into the mix, the tension between the functional and spirit views of power could be reconciled. The two poles can be transcended and included; both can be framed as an *and* through the being dimension.

Relevance of Phenomenological Scholarship to My Life and Work

A major understanding from my findings is that personal power, in its essence, is a lived experience in one's being. From my protocol analysis, I found that my being was the medium for my will to be expressed in my doing at the functional level. Power is presented nearly exclusively as some quantity or possession. It is viewed generally as something one either has or does not have, like money or weight. It is presented most often as a one-dimensional phenomenon. I have found these presentations of power are not wrong, but incomplete. As a lived experience, power is multidimensional and complex. Any understanding of power must account for personal experience. My findings offer a different way to look at the literature of power. A hermeneutic-phenomenological perspective on power challenges the definitions and claims of the prevailing rational-empirical perspectives on power.

My study has added significant value to my life, and the lives of others, through its use in my consulting business. At the personal level, the application of my learning from my research holds the ongoing promise of helping me to realize more of my potential *to be* and *to do*. My study has been a significant transitional event in my life in a number of ways. As a result of my inquiry, my beliefs in many areas have changed. My ability as a consultant has been enhanced. I have discovered and started to develop an aspect of my voice that I did not realize I had. I have learned to have greater trust in my self, and that I will always have power because I always have a choice in any situation.

My study has also led to additional revenue generation and work satisfaction in my consulting business. Using both the process and outcomes of my inquiry, I developed a unique executive/management development program entitled *Higher Order Thinking (HOT) Program: Mastering Executive Power*. The first level of the HOT Program is five full days of group sessions, spread over a four-month period, with monthly individual coaching in between the group sessions. Each group consists of eight to ten executives or senior managers from the corporate, public service, and not-for-profit sectors. Participants are guided through their own inquiry into their peak power experiences, in much the same way that I did my inquiry into my experiences, but on a smaller and more simplified scale. They share their experiences, extract their own insights, and discuss how to embody their findings into their lives. Through a process of Socratic dialogue, they are guided through modules of higher order conceptual frameworks such as Bennett's systematics. They apply these frameworks over the four-month period on projects significant to them.

My aim in this chapter has been to walk briskly through a decade of my life inquiry into power. My hope is that, by reading this chapter, you will reflect on your experience of power and gain a deeper appreciation of the practical utility of hermeneutic phenomenology.

REFERENCES

Ahl, Valerie, and Timothy F. H. Allen. (1996) *Hierarchy Theory: A Vision, Vocabulary, and Epistemology.* New York: Columbia University Press.

Bennett, John G. (1993) *Elementary Systematics: A Tool for Understanding Wholes.* Santa Fe, NM: Bennett Books.

———. (1994) *Deeper Man*. Santa Fe, NM: Bennett Books.

———. (1997) *The Dramatic Universe: Vol. III. Man and His Nature*. Charles Town, WV: Claymont Communications.

Bentz, Valerie M. (1989) *Becoming Mature: Childhood Ghosts and Spirits in Adult Life*. Hawthorne, NY: Aldine de Gruyter.

Bentz, Valerie M., and Jeremy J. Shapiro. (1998) *Mindful Inquiry in Social Research*. London: Sage.

Gadamer, Hans-Georg. (1975) *Truth and Method*. New York: Continuum.

Husserl, Edmund. (1970) *The Crisis of European Sciences and Transcendental Phenomenology*. Evanston, IL: Northwestern University Press.

Mintzberg, Henry. (1983) *Power In and Around Organizations*. Englewood Cliffs, NJ: Prentice-Hall.

Novokowsky, Bernie J. (1999) *Personal Power: The Realization of Doing and Being*. Unpublished Ph.D. Dissertation, Santa Barbara, CA: Fielding Graduate Institute.

Simon, Herbert A. (1973) The Organization of Complex Systems. In H. H. Pattee (Ed.), *Hierarchy Theory: The Challenge of Complex Systems*. New York: George Braziller.

van Manen, Max. (1990) *Researching Lived Experience*. London, Ontario, Canada: The Althouse Press.

9

Bodymindfulness and Energetic Presence in Intercultural Communication

Adair Linn Nagata

PHENOMENOLOGICAL PRACTICE AT WORK

> Human resource professionals who work with people of many nationalities and traditions outside their own culture face a similar challenge whether their company is multinational, international, transnational or global. Few of us have achieved a worldcentric level of consciousness and the requisite skills for managing our relationships according to the human resource policies that many of our companies have now mandated. Many of us work for organizations that base promotion and compensation on performance and merit. These policies are intended to be applied globally in spite of local practices that are based on antithetical assumptions and traditions and despite our own possible quirks of mind and manner that may be out of the awareness of those of us who are entrusted with administering them. (Nagata, 1998, 143)

The preceding passage summarizes my reflections on the special learning opportunity I had every day at work in the Japanese offices of a financial services firm with operations in one hundred countries. When I first began doing organizational development work in Japan, I imagined that my central task would be to promote a family-friendly workplace, one that would shift the mindset of middle managers away from their global motto of *never sleeps*. Finding how to do this entailed a need for watchfulness, especially a need to understand how communications worked.

I carefully observed myself and other people in regard to bodily cues for quite some time, and realized that our bodies hold us in positions that affect our ability to accept and utilize new ideas or realities in our work environments. I could see, hear, and feel tension, muscular contraction, and postural stiffening when new policies and programs were announced and managers were still uncomfortable with the idea or the effort that implementing them would require. I came to the realization that organizational change could only happen if it emerged from and encompassed the *body-mindset* of the personnel—their existing patterns of being in their body-minds. This insight became one of the bases for my doctoral research work, one that led to a transformation of my self-awareness and my approach to practicing and later teaching intercultural communication (Nagata, 2002, 2007).

In this essay, I describe how my background as a USAmerican living and working in Japan drew me to see that a new conception—*bodymindfulness of bodymindset*—was needed to account for and foster change within Japanese middle managers. In pursuit of research stemming from my workplace realization, I discovered and was changed by entry into the phenomenological domain of inquiry. While phenomenology provided the methodology for my research purposes, working within this domain shifted my awareness of self and eventually transformed all of my work in the area of intercultural communication.

DISTURBING THE *WA*: A USAMERICAN IN JAPAN

I learned the hard way about the famous Japanese sense of harmony called *wa*, because I seemed to have had a talent for disturbing it. As a well-educated European–USAmerican who came to live and work in Japan in 1970 when already a young adult, I lacked a common linguistic or cultural background to rely upon as I struggled to gain emotional and communicative competence in my new culture. Without the ability to communicate well in words, read Japanese characters, or decode unfamiliar cultural cues, I repeatedly found myself beyond my experience, out of my depth, often teetering at the edge of my ability to make sense of what was happening around me, or losing my balance and regretting how I handled myself.

In the discordant situations I experienced in my new life, I found myself becoming more and more aware of my internal states, the prelinguistic, somatic (body experienced from within) ground of the linguistic competence I was lacking (see Behnke, 1997). I recognized that I needed a way to calm myself, gain perspective, and continue trying to deal with whatever or whomever I found perplexing. In addition to the challenges of family life in an international marriage, my paid employment had been in international education, and later in corporate human resources, at what I call the *intercultural interface*, where people of diverse cultures live and work together (see Nagata, 1998). I have had a long internship in learning about the necessity for bodily sensitivity as the basis for relational attunement, which I came to call *embodied empathic resonance.* I felt considerable need to create harmony in and around me as I tried to learn about *interbeing*—the deep relational interconnectedness between people—in the group-oriented culture where I now make my home (see Nhat Hanh, 1996).

During my doctoral studies, undertaken after twenty-six years in Japan, I pursued what Bentz and Shapiro (1998) call *mindful inquiry,* applying it to the deeper relational skills that I recognized were needed in my life in my second culture. I kept an ongoing journal of my experiences over the next several years. In trying to understand how Japanese people seemed to sense the atmosphere and communicate without words, I discovered the power and value of *bodymindfulness*—a term I coined for attending to somatic sensations and their relation to thought and feeling. I learned to attune to *energetic presence*—a person's living presence and the message it communicates, whether or not the person is conscious of it (Nagata, 2002; Palmer, 1999).

PHENOMENOLOGY AND THE LIVED EXPERIENCE OF INTERCULTURAL COMMUNICATION

Intercultural communication prepared me to do phenomenology, and phenomenology deepened my ability to relate, especially interculturally. The continual discipline of observing and trying to make sense of my intercultural interactions has been a kind of phenomenological training. Every day, I have been confronted with my USAmerican cultural assumptions, and I have had to learn to suspend them, and often what I thought I understood about Japan as well. Living in Japan exposed me to traditions that do not make the same distinctions regarding mind, body, and self as those with which I was raised. I pursued Asian body/mind practices, such as tai chi and *kikou* (Chinese energy healing), that continue to help me experience increasing integration of the multiple realms of being: body, emotion/feeling, mind, and spirit. These efforts required a bracketing or suspension of some of my assumptions.

The most important assumption related to this inquiry is the one that Alan Watts addresses in *The Book: On the Taboo Against Knowing Who You Are:* "The prevalent sensation of oneself as a separate ego enclosed in a bag of skin is a hallucination which accords neither with Western science nor with the experimental philosophy-religions of the East" (1966, ix). I was raised to believe that I was an autonomous individual, responsible for myself, and that the purpose of my education was to cultivate my unique potential. I assumed the subject-object model of relationships. As a young girl growing up in the 1950s (before I ever became aware of feminism), I determinedly pursued being taken seriously as a subject. I only developed a tacit understanding of intersubjectivity, how our relationships impact us, slowly, through reflection on endless relational difficulties. At that time, sharing of vital energy between people was not easily imaginable. Sustained personal consciousness of the interconnection of all life was even more difficult to contemplate.

At the beginning of my studies, I had to figure out what I needed to understand about Japanese relational and communication skills, and then I had to work to understand it. Virtually all aspects of my life contributed to my inquiry. For six years of doctoral study, I was immersed in these efforts, literally day and night, as working with my dreams had been part of my personal practice for years. All my activities and attempts to figure out how to be a more appropriate, effective, and satisfied communicator in my adopted culture had a seamless quality, and phenomenology continually helped me to bring more aspects of my lived experience into awareness. Most of my daily encounters could provoke reflection in my journals, if I were lucky enough to have the time to express them in writing. More typically, I just had to think quickly on my feet. As a result, I have developed a high degree of reflexivity: "To be reflexive is to have an ongoing conversation about experience while simultaneously living in the moment" (Hertz, 1997, viii).

Intercultural interactions necessitated this ability to reflect in the here and now, and the practice of phenomenological writing helped me to cultivate a similar sort of consciousness for use in the midst of my daily encounters. Self-reflexivity, the ability to understand ourselves and our position in society, is considered an ethical necessity for interculturalists (Martin and Nakayama, 2007, 36). Interculturalists are persons who are dedicated to communicating effectively across cultural boundaries and oriented to examining their own assumptions, values, and behaviors to enlarge their own relational abilities. Self-reflexivity is my personal aspiration and the thrust of my current university teaching as a professor of intercultural communication.

Using phenomenology for my multilayered inquiry into the self was most illuminating. The reflecting I have done in writing was preparation for doing the epoche, phenomenological reduction, imaginative variation, and synthesis of phenomenology (Moustakas, 1994). Repeated efforts to bracket my assumptions and use imaginative variations helped me to consider other alternatives. Interviewing twelve other interculturalists further increased my awareness of my assumptions. Their lived experiences both validated and suggested alternatives to my own construals and choices. Continually distilling of what I was finding as I did phenomenological reduction and synthesizing everything into a description promoted increased awareness.

PUTTING PHENOMENOLOGY TO WORK

Two years before I retired from corporate life in Japan, my work role changed; I became a designated change agent in the human resources department. My new responsibilities were to customize so-called *global* human resource policies and programs that promoted work/life balance for use in a country, language, and culture different from where they were formulated. I recognized that I, as a phenomenologist, became an instrument of change in this new role and would be changed in the process. I wrote about the most interesting encounters of the day in as much detail as I could remember. The insights I gained from this reflective practice were responsible for my being able to function at a heightened level of courage and confidence.

As a change agent championing workplace satisfaction, I needed to create openings for consideration of unfamiliar concepts, labor law changes, and proposed new policies and programs, and hold space open to unprecedented experience—situations involving human intricacy and uncertainty—while promoting their acceptance and utilization. My personal challenge was keeping myself open to what was unfolding in conversations and meetings, while simultaneously trying to maintain this required new direction.

Developing a New Guide

Attending to messages from my body/mind promoted its further integration by moving me beyond what I came to call the *bodymindset*—my existing pattern of being in my body/mind. Trust in the deep knowing of our body/mind builds confidence, because it is readily available, although subconscious, and can be quickly utilized simply by being present to it (see Pert, 2000). The body/mind mediates inner experiences and outer circumstances, guiding alignment with the flow of the situation. Bodymindfulness arises from the combined processing of somatic-emotional and cognitive information into an enlarged, integrated form of intelligence that became indispensable in my practice. This intelligence can be engaged by sensing the *inner aura*—Gendlin's term for the felt sense of a person, object, situation, or idea (1981, 53–54)—of our own energetic presence, that of others in the interaction, and/or the atmosphere pervading the situation.

As I became more attentive to the internal states of my body/mind, I began to use it as an instrument to guide me in my efforts to connect with other people. I became interested in the energetic, vibratory aspects of interpersonal interactions that are nonverbal and often beyond awareness. I came to use the phrase *embodied empathic resonance* to reflect both the aspects of somatic-emotional experience and of interpersonal connection in what transpersonal psychologist Ken Wilber terms *common emotional world-space* (1996, 99). Insight into managing the bodymindset came from attempts to manage my own. The more I attended to somatic-emotional feelings, the more I noticed the energetic presence of people as they greeted and interacted with me. Important differences in nonverbal styles of cultures manifest most clearly in greetings, status differences, communication of emotions, and intimacy (Leathers, 1997). Attending to these with body-mindfulness became a rich source of relational insights.

I discovered, by observing myself and interpersonal interactions, that good timing is a function of sensitivity to embodied empathic resonance. When I needed to work with a colleague, I would approach his desk and stand and wait without saying anything until he gave me his attention. Sometimes, when it was obvious that the person was too busy to attend productively to what I needed in the time available, I withdrew without saying anything. When it was clear that someone with whom I was interacting was not existentially present and attentive, I learned to change my approach. If possible, I offered to come back or have the conversation at another time. Consideration for others' work demands and pace helped to build collaborative relationships. Then, when I had to be insistent, I could usually gain cooperation, because the person knew that it was truly urgent. My work in formulating policy and programs related to work/life balance, and the preparation of the employee communication and training materials involved interviewing managers and interested employees. Interviewing two male managers, separately, but during the same time period, for one project made me particularly conscious of how flexible I needed to be in order to match the pace and communication style of the person I was interviewing.

The two men exemplified different communicative ideals typical of their native cultures, USAmerican and Japanese: Mr. A. was highly articulate, a persuasive talker; Mr. J. was a careful listener, whose sensitive cueing to me during conversation influenced what he would say. If I had not been quick, expressive, and highly flexible, I would not even have been able to schedule the interview with Mr. A., much less hold his attention. If I had been impatient or critical with Mr. J., he would not have shared the anecdotes that gave me insights into what really goes on in a Japanese work group. If I had not sensed, nonverbally, when to wait and when to move on, he probably would have given me much less detail. By selectively clarifying things that he said without a judgmental tone, I may have been able to extend his thinking into less familiar territory. That was my interpretation of his comment at the end: that he had found the interview surprisingly interesting and useful. Experiences like these helped me to recognize that the communicative flexibility required in my work was based in bodymindfulness and sensitivity to energetic presence.

Heightening Awareness Empowers Skillful Choices

Developing greater sensitivity does not just heighten feelings of success and pleasure. I had to monitor myself carefully so that I did not overreact when I felt slighted. In a series of interactions with Japanese male managers, who were seemingly unaccustomed to working with senior women officers, I found that, by writing about the incidents afterward, my somatic sense of boundary violation had protectively alerted me to the need to shift my bodymindset to demonstrate the need for greater respect. The following is one example.

> Today I had an appointment with Mr. H., our new HR generalist, which was intended for us to get to know each other in order to facilitate our work together. When I changed not long ago to working only 60 percent, I moved from my large office in the training center to the smallest size carrel in the HR department proper upstairs; so I went to his spacious office for our meeting. He was not there, and I returned to my desk for more than twenty minutes before I was informed that he had returned and would see me. He did not apologize for keeping me waiting, and I felt myself contract and become wary and cooler in manner than I had felt when I had originally gone to his office at the appointed time in eager anticipation of our first meeting.

I observed the shift in my orientation to my colleague when I felt disrespected and sensed dissonance both within myself and between us.

> As we talked, he must have realized my long years of service and varied experiences in the company could be quite helpful to him in projects that we were expected to do together. My usual style is collaborative and supportive, but I was quite formal and matter of fact and interacted without much eye contact or warmth. I also did not do the amount of verbal and nonverbal interaction work typically expected of women.

The content and style of what I communicated to him seemed to have contributed to his realization that I deserved his interest and his respect.

> By the end of our conversation forty minutes later, he spontaneously apologized for keeping me waiting, and I nodded my acceptance. Somehow I elicited this spontaneous apology, a real rarity from a senior Japanese man. In addition to his apparent lack of experience working with foreign women managers, I surmise that his behavior is typically hierarchical; and he was probably judging from my workspace that I was his inferior when in actuality I was his superior in corporate rank and age as well as experience in the company. (Journal, April 23, 1999)

On later occasions when my time or contribution did not seem to have been valued, I was more aware as I monitored the irritation I felt. I was more able to choose how much to allow it to leak out and be read and accommodated by a sensitive Japanese counterpart. My self-presentation through energetic presence would shift, especially posture and movements, eye contact, and use of voice. As I became more skillful, I would get the information I needed from somatic-emotional feelings, act on them, and then let them go, so that there was minimal unfinished business between us that would affect future dealings.

When my writing revealed what had been happening, I felt that it reflected my changing sense of confidence and emergent personal power, as I increasingly trusted my body/mind to guide me. Using the phenomenological strategy of writing protocols (descriptions like the one above) about these interactions made me aware of the shifts that had occurred unintentionally. These realizations then enabled me to choose consciously to alter my behavior. The cyclical process of writing, reading, and rewriting the descriptions of such experiences helped me to see patterns and themes that contributed to a knowing that gave me new confidence.

Everyday Peacemaking

As my mindful inquiry progressed, I developed more bodymindfulness and sensitivity to the somatic tonality of energetic presence. At the same time, my understanding of consonance and dissonance was growing, and I did not find it so necessary to minimize differences of opinion or avoid conflict, which had been my tendency. I was able to contribute to dealing with conflicts more comfortably and productively, sometimes moving them toward mutually agreeable resolution, that is, to practice everyday peacemaking both within and around me. *Everyday peacemaking* is acting wherever we find ourselves to reduce inequality and promote understanding (Chambliss, 2002).

Initially, I was not intentionally attempting to provide a calming presence, but I consciously began to try if it seemed that this would be welcome. Sometimes, when someone else was upset, it was possible for me to be very centered, be present, and follow the flow of his energy. I tried to hold myself open and listen to what he was concerned about. Gradually, as the person's emotional temperature subsided, we were able to discuss alternative views or possible actions. This has become the most common form of everyday peacemaking in which I engage.

A conversation over lunch with a woman senior executive shows the effect that being centered can have on the other person. This vignette from corporate life includes awareness of bodymindset and energetic presence that are effective preparation for real-time multinational power dynamics.

I had lunch with Ms. S. today and we talked about self-management when your boss is being verbally abusive, especially in front of other people. She had just

come from a weekly meeting involving senior managers of around five nationalities. She said she could tell that her boss was very stressed when he
walked in and that he would beat up on everyone in turn except a few men
who are his favorites. She said she felt fear this morning. She tries to stay centered and respond very professionally, taking responsibility without blaming
or cringing. She said she could see him holding himself back from going any
further with her even though he wanted to. She observed that she sometimes
feels stubborn, but I said I thought that not allowing oneself to be knocked off
center can be a positive aspect of centering.

Ms. S. observed her boss as he came through the door and got ready to hold
herself to her professional standards, expecting to be under fire from his
verbal abuse. Even a small lead-time on the communications challenge she
had to face helped her to maintain balance and not respond in kind. Both
her self-management in the incident she reported and how I tried to witness
her story suggest what I term *coherent energy*, a deep physiologically based
centeredness that can affect those around us.

> She has found ways of calming herself internally when she begins to feel over-
> whelmed. Sometimes she calls her husband and they have lunch and never
> speak about business. Sometimes she goes home early and gets a good night's
> sleep. I think that her bodily awareness serves her well and provides bound-
> aries that protect her and model a better way than fighting back which just es-
> calates. I encouraged her, saying that the other people in the meeting also ben-
> efit from seeing the different example she sets and may learn from how she
> handles herself. She said our lunch conversation was a blessing as she had be-
> come more conscious of some of the things she does and felt much better than
> she had at the end of the stressful meeting. (Journal, November 28, 2000)

I was glad to hear, not long afterward, that she had been promoted into her
boss's job. I thought again how practical applying understanding of embodied empathic resonance can be.

Cultivating Bodymindfulness

In my new career as a university educator, I begin with a seemingly simple exercise that I call the *bodymindfulness practice*. It promotes development
of awareness of our bodymindset and offers a means of shifting it so that
our energetic presence is more poised and effective in conveying a desired
message congruently. Here are the steps:

- Presence requires being present in the moment: *Be here now.*
- Tune into your breathing and see what it tells you about your current
  state of being.
- Breathe more deeply and evenly.

- Set your intention for your participation.
- Use bodymindfulness to be here now!

The bodymindfulness practice is intended as a means of attuning to our bodily feelings, diagnosing our internal state, and then changing it if desirable. It is a distillation of Asian practices that can be done anytime, anywhere, at no cost, and in the complete privacy of one's own body/mind. No one else needs to know that it is needed or being performed. I encourage my students to make it a regular practice by doing it each time they enter a room and/or engage with someone. The intention is that, eventually, this process of self-attunement will pass out of awareness and become an automatic response. Student reflections on their experiences of learning and applying bodymindfulness have revealed how they responded with enhanced self-awareness, improved communication skills, and new ways of being and doing (Nagata, 2007).

PHENOMENOLOGICAL DESCRIPTION OF EMBODIED EMPATHIC RESONANCE

Based on my own journals and descriptions, along with in-depth interviews of twelve highly functioning interculturalists, I developed a concise understanding of the nature and dimensions of the phenomenon of *embodied empathic resonance* (Nagata, 2002). The participants in my research are men and women of six nationalities, who have collectively lived and worked in more than thirty-five countries. I present here a concise formulation of the new understanding that emerged from using phenomenology and hermeneutics as part of my practice.

Embodied empathic resonance is the body/mind's experience of energetic vibration from both internal (vital pulses such as brain waves, breath, and heart rate) and external (other living bodies, machines, and the macrocosm) sources. Two levels of functioning in face-to-face interactions provide a means of empathic relational attunement that is the basis for mutuality:

1. *Intrapersonal*: Integration of body, mind, and spirit creates a consonant state in which energy flows freely in the present within our total being, and we have a sense of being authentic and acting with synergetic access to our internal resources. Blockages, splits, separations, disconnections, and disruption of energy flow are evidence of and contribute to dissonant states that have opposite characteristics.

2. *Interpersonal*: Authentic interactions in face-to-face relationships are those in which we are able to be present, express ourselves, and tune in and respond to another, so that a mutually satisfying connection

can be made if it is deemed desirable. In dissonant interactions, connection is not made in a deeply satisfying way, and this often provides motivation for change.

Embodied empathic resonance is the basis of a somatic way of knowing that includes somatic-emotional sensations and the felt sense, the inner aura of the energetic presence of our own being or that of another in states ranging from dissonance to consonance. Dissonant states grab our attention and are generally more noticeable. Bodymindfulness of the experience of energetic presence, either dissonant or consonant, can enable us to relate more skillfully.

Bodymindfulness needs to be cultivated in order to be able to attune to our inner states and those of the people with whom we are relating. *Bodymindfulness* is my term for attending to bodily and emotional sensations and associated thoughts, including those of the other person(s), during interpersonal interactions. Bodymindfulness is an intrapersonal component of embodiment. Attending to the flow of our internal states with equanimity is a powerful tool for self-knowledge and a transformative discipline with significant relational effects (Young, 1997).

Consonance and dissonance are the harmonious and discordant ends of the spectrum of resonant emotional experience. Resonance provides the connection for the emotion of verbal or nonverbal communication. Resonant emotional connections can range from comfortable and welcome to uncomfortable, even upsetting. Making this distinction and understanding the phenomenon of embodied empathic resonance can enhance our relational skills because we can be more conscious of what is happening, especially in emotionally charged encounters. Typical consonant experiences are comfortable, smooth, and characterized by relaxation, flow, and often a sense of prior knowing.

Dissonant experiences are characterized sometimes by a lack of connection that may result in disappointment and low energy, at least on the side of the hopeful or needful party. Extremely dissonant encounters may be highly energized engagements where people experience a similar dissonant state such as anger and/or feel strong aversion to each other's energetic presences. Cutoffs, refusals by someone to interact with particular people or groups, may be explained partially by the somatic-emotional distress that being in their presence may engender.

Intense states of either consonance or dissonance are highly resonant and, yin/yang-like, may shift from one into the other when they reach fullness. Understanding this complementarity and using compassion can promote this movement into relational connections even when the prevailing effect has been disturbing. This is the motivating hope of everyday peacemaking.

Shifting the bodymindset is a somatic epistemology, or way of knowing, for managing our emotional energy to work with our internal state, protect our safety, and/or improve our relationships. Working with my phenomenological protocols, I identified six themes in shifting the bodymindset and arranged them to build on one another:

1. Opening myself to the full range of resonant relational possibilities from consonance to dissonance;
2. Feeling and holding with whatever comes, including not knowing;
3. Clarifying whether the emotional energy is primarily internally generated or a resonant echo of someone else's emotional state;
4. Being authentic in the flow of the moment and trusting the process;
5. Shifting and releasing after getting and using the information; and
6. Claiming personal power and moving forward.

This six-step approach to shifting the bodymindset functions on both the intrapersonal and interpersonal levels. In my current university teaching and intercultural training courses, I now teach *shifting the bodymindset* with the intention of empowering people who want to improve their relational skills. Through my pursuit of mindful inquiry, I experienced greater openness, fluidity, and trust. This enhanced my work as an internal organizational consultant and took me beyond that which I had thought I was capable. My whole being was absorbed in this inquiry, so that I reached a new level of embodied understanding and found myself embodying these changes in action.

REFLECTING ON THE POWER OF PHENOMENOLOGY

My path of change led to an appreciation of a somatically enhanced epistemology that I can trust. Practicing phenomenology and hermeneutics promoted my personal and professional development. I began to work at the edge of my capabilities without becoming exhausted and unproductive. I created greater work/life balance in my own life, which my colleagues told me served as a model for them.

Although living in Tokyo can be spatially and psychically restrictive for a non-Japanese woman, it has been a valuable framework for learning and self-mastery. In "Learning at the Margin: New Models of Strength," Judith Jordan (2000) reinterprets the value of an outsider position as increasing consciousness and affording perspective and access to alternative versions of truth. During my many years in Japan, I have been learning how to construct a satisfying life on the margin of Japanese society; and Jordan's view accords with my own positive evaluation of this positioning. I aspire to what Janet Bennett terms *constructive marginality* (1993). I have become aware that peace, both inner and outer, is essential for my life to continue along this fulfilling path. I might not have attained this clarity without having pursued a phenomenological practice.

Phenomenological work helped me to be in touch with my body/mind's innate ability to intuit in order to be a sensitive and effective communicator with diverse people in fluid situations. It gave me access to an elusive and wordless phenomenon and led me to understand how embodied empathic resonance as a prelinguistic source of information can guide us in relationships. It enabled me to comprehend how bodymindfulness of embodied empathic resonance can be especially valuable in relating to all people, especially those who we believe are significantly different from ourselves, even if we may not share a common language.

Differences are often seen as problematic: the cause of separation, the flashpoint for aggression, the source of dissonance and suffering. This is especially the case in Japan. I now consider encounter with differences as an invitation to develop higher awareness through intrapersonal and interpersonal work, an opportunity to increase consciousness and enlarge our sense of humanity and personal humanness. Working with dissonance created by differences can lead toward authentic connections, both within and between people. Dissonance grabs attention and, when attended to in the body and processed with compassion, can become an impetus to personal growth and social change. For me, one of the most positive aspects of differences—cultural, gender, or any other kind—is their potential for expanding awareness and increasing consciousness. Phenomenology and hermeneutics are the perfect tools for describing and interpreting differences of all kinds.

REFERENCES

Behnke, Elizabeth. (1997) Somatics. In L. Embree (Adapt.), *Encyclopedia of Phenomenology* (663–67). Dordrecht, The Netherlands: Kluwer Academic.

Bennett, Janet M. (1993) Cultural Marginality: Identity Issues in Intercultural Training. In R. M. Paige, *Education for the Intercultural Experience* (109–35). Yarmouth, ME: Intercultural Press.

Bentz, Valerie M., and Jeremy J. Shapiro. (1998) *Mindful Inquiry in Social Research.* Thousand Oaks, CA: Sage.

Chambliss, Barbara B. (2002) *Contemporary Women Peacemakers: The Hidden Side of Peacemaking.* Unpublished Ph.D. Dissertation. Santa Barbara, CA: Fielding Graduate Institute.

Gendlin, Eugene T. (1981) *Focusing* (second ed.). New York: Bantam.

Hertz, Rosanna (Ed.). (1997) *Reflexivity and Voice.* Thousand Oaks, CA: Sage.

Jordan, Judith V. (2000) Learning at the Margin: New Models of Strength. *Work in Progress* (No. 98). Wellesley, MA: Stone Center Working Paper Series.

Leathers, Dale G. (1997) *Successful Nonverbal Communication: Principles and Applications* (third ed.). Boston: Allyn & Bacon.

Martin, Judith N., and Thomas K. Nakayama. (2007) *Intercultural Communication in Contexts* (fourth ed.). New York: McGraw-Hill.

Moustakas, Clark. (1994) *Phenomenological Research Methods*. Thousand Oaks, CA: Sage.

Nagata, Adair L. (1998) Being Global: Life at the Interface. *Human Resource Development International, 1*(2), 143–45.

———. (2002) Somatic Mindfulness and Energetic Presence in Intercultural Communication: A Phenomenological/Hermeneutic Exploration of Bodymindset and Emotional Resonance. Unpublished Ph.D. Dissertation. Santa Barbara, CA: Fielding Graduate Institute.

———. (2007) Bodymindfulness for Skillful Communication. *Intercultural Communication Review, 5*, 61–76.

Nhat Hanh, Thich. (1996) *Being Peace*. Berkeley, CA: Parallax Press.

Palmer, Wendy. (1999) *The Intuitive Body: Aikido as a Clairsentient Practice* (Rev. ed.). Berkeley, CA: North Atlantic Books.

Pert, Candace B. (2000) *Your Body Is Your Subconscious Mind* [cassette recordings]. Boulder, CO: Sounds True.

Watts, Alan. (1966) *The Book: On the Taboo Against Knowing Who You Are*. New York: Pantheon Books.

Wilber, Ken. (1996) *A Brief History of Everything*. Boston: Shambhala.

Young, Shinzen. (1997) *The Science of Enlightenment: Teachings and Meditations for Awakening Through Self-Investigation* [cassette recordings]. Boulder, CO: Sounds True.

IV

EXPERIENCING TRANSCENDENCE: PERSONAL TRANSFORMATION AS COLLABORATIVE ACCOMPLISHMENT

10

Finding Voice and Reclaiming Identity

Embodied Wisdom in the Lived Experience of Norteñas de Nuevo Méjico

Gloria L. Córdova

In my hermeneutic-phenomenological research study, a group of northern New Mexico Latinas shared rich descriptions of their lives. They allowed me to explore and analyze their life stories in order to recover a sense of lost voice and reclaim their identity. I, too, am a Latina from northern New Mexico. Their narratives provided the opportunity to discern and build *theory in the flesh* (Aquino, Machado, and Rodriguez, 2002, xiv–iv; Moraga and Anzaldúa, 1983). Conducting the study was a transformational experience for me and for them. It also changed my professional practice from human resource development to consciousness development.

I begin this chapter by providing an historical sketch to personalize Latinas and our unique ancestry. I then discuss six themes as elements of the essence of the northern New Mexico Latina lived experience in finding voice and claiming identity. Next, I analyze consciousness development as a nascent theory of the *conscientización*. I conclude with a brief discussion of my own learning to recognize and deal with my own internalized oppression and to reclaim pride in my ethnic and cultural roots.

HISTORICAL CONTEXTUALIZATION: THE LATINAS OF NORTHERN NEW MEXICO

The Latinas who shared their stories are geographically, culturally, and historically a unique group of women. Understanding our history and identity is necessary to the interpretation of our experience (de la Torre and Pesquera, 1993). The story of our ancestry recalls that Spanish colonizers discovered America and the civilizations of its indigenous peoples. Spanish soldiers settled in what is now northern New Mexico in the early sixteenth century, colonizing and racially mixing with these people and their descendants. Mexican women became United States citizens by default in 1848 after the U.S.-Mexican War. The border literally *migrated to them*, imposing a foreign language and socio-legal system. Following the 1848 Treaty of Guadalupe-Hidalgo, our historical story speaks of displacement from our land (Ebright, 1994; E. Martinez, 1995), the acceptance of political-economic dependence on an industrial society (Briggs, 1999), and disenfranchisement and segregation (Zavella, 1991).

We are the descendants of those women of Spanish, Mexican, and Native American heritage, known today by a variety of names, including Hispanas, Spanish-Americans, Mexican-Americans, Latinas, Chicanas, and *mestizas*, racially mixed European, and American Indian. Within the context of my research, the women who participated are, more specifically, the northern New Mexico descendants of Spanish-Mexican–Native American women. We live and have ancestral family *nativo* roots in what is, today, northern New Mexico, forged by our ancestors, who settled as early as 1595 (Esquibel, 1998). Others, who were not here with the original settlers, come from families that were long settled in the land when the northern frontier of Mexico became a territory of the United States. Our ancestors founded families whose surnames are in the family lines of Latino people in New Mexico today (Esquibel and Preston, 1998). Our cultural roots are long-standing.

The change to a territory after 1848, and later statehood, left the majority of Spanish-Mexican citizens in New Mexico, particularly the women, impoverished and in low-paid labor. This trend persists today (Gonzalez, 1999). The women in this study were born and raised in the fallout of the political-economic history that relegated our families to a lower class, and objectified us through insidious stereotyping of our culture; our cultural heritage is seen as limiting our educational, social, or political potentialities, a culture-determined notion of *blaming the victim* (Zavella, 1991, 75–76).

The study participants are Latinas who, to varying degrees, reclaimed and reconstructed our lives and senses of self, despite the many forms of continuing subordination. Even today, Latinas live with the consequences of the mechanisms that institutionalized oppression, racism, sexism, and working-class status, which evolved from the colonization of our antecedent families, into North American society (Zavella, 1991). For hegemony to be preserved, the experiences of the oppressed must remain invisible. A central goal of my study was to make those experiences visible and explicit.

DISSONANCE AND CONSONANCE WITHIN THEMES
FROM THE WOMEN'S NARRATIVES

The research was conducted over the years 2000 to 2002, and involved eight Latinas, including myself, who self-identified and volunteered to participate in the study. The women ranged in age from late forties to mid-sixties. They agreed to be audiotaped in a series of several-hour-long, open-ended, in-depth interviews. The names used here are pseudonyms. Selections from the participants' narratives illustrate six themes of our lived experience, noting dissonance and consonance within each theme. The selected quotations display the women learning to recognize and deal with internalized oppression, which they each experienced as a result of dissonant experiences over a lifetime. In the conclusion of this essay, one can better understand how the Latinas experienced personal discovery and developed self-understanding and improved self-esteem.

I identified dissonance and consonance in six core themes common to all participants (Córdova, 2004). There were two sides to each of the themes of lived experience, as summarized in table 10.1.

Spanish as a First Language: Theme 1

> *Stella*: When I went to first grade, I couldn't speak English because I spoke Spanish at home. So I had to learn how to speak English. I've always been bilingual since then, but I've always been very careful about my English. I remember in grade school a teacher made me write one hundred times on the board [here Stella emphasized the letter "C"]: "C-H-I-N-A" because I pronounced the "c" like an "s," saying "Shina."

This shame affects Stella even today. Her speech lilts with a lovely cadence, inflection, and rhythm, typical in the speech pattern of *nativos* of northern New Mexico. She does not hear that her speech sounds different from non-natives; she does not want to be heard as speaking with a distinguishable accent.

Nevertheless, the Latinas whose first language was Spanish all indicated that they now are grateful that they are bilingual. Teresa beautifully expressed her sense of appreciation of her native language:

> *Teresa*: I think [speaking Spanish] has always been a very rich experience, [even] more so as I get older, [because] I realize that I see things from two points of view most of the time. And in a way that gives you a lot more material to work with. I know we have a lot of . . . wisdom.

Table 10.1. Topics and Emergent Themes From the Latinas' Experience

Topics	Themes			Sources of the Latinas' Experience
	Dissonant	and	Consonant	
Language	Handicap	and	Gift	Spanish or English as a first language
Religion	Ritual and religiosity rejected	and	Faith and spirituality claimed	Religion in family and culture
Education	Opportunity lost	and	Opportunity gained	Attitudes toward and prospects for education in family and society
Skin color	Wound	and	Blessing	Attitudes toward fair (*güera*) and dark (*prieta*) skin color within family and society
Family and relationships	Wound	and	Blessing	Family and relationships
Ethnic identity	Pain and anger of oppression	and	Blessing and pride in heritage	Ethnic identity and consciousness development

Note. From *The Lived Experience of Norteñas de Nuevo Méjico: Finding Voice and Reclaiming Identity* (unpublished doctoral dissertation, pp. 71-72), by G. L. Córdova, 2004, Santa Barbara, CA: Fielding Graduate Institute. Copyright 2004 by Gloria L. Córdova. Adapted by the author.

These examples illustrate the dissonance (handicap) and consonance (gift) in the Latinas' experience of Spanish as a first language.

Religion: Theme 2

As with language, religion also drew out themes of dissonance—ritual and religiosity rejected—and consonance—faith and spirituality claimed. Dissonant experiences were often connected with memories of being raised Catholic. Stella spoke animatedly about her memories of being raised in the Catholic faith tradition, as practiced in her home:

Stella: Well, we used to go to church every Sunday when we were little kids, you know. And we got pinched if we whispered something. [Stella made a sound indicating reprimand.] "What! Be quiet." Mom would go like that down the line from the oldest one to the youngest. I used to hate for her to do it, you know. And, I mean, we were in church a lot! We used to say the rosary and kneel down at home. We used to get the *Sagrada Familia* [sacred family, a statue that traveled from home to home]; you know. My mom and my grandma belonged to the Society [people of a parish belonged to the Society of the *Sagrada Familia*]. So whenever we had the *Sagrada Familia*, we would pray as a family— my grandma and my grandpa, and my cousins, and us, you know, our whole family—and then they'd go on and on and on.

All these prayers! Like, how could they memorize all those prayers? And, of course, they're all in Spanish. And we were just there [kneeling] on the linoleum floor, the wood floor, and I'm like, "Oh, my gosh!" And the minute you'd kind of go like this [Stella gestured as though she was restless or weary], they'd pinch you or they go like that [Stella gestured again], "Kneel up. Kneel straight!"

While Stella described a dissonant experience with religion, ending with her rejection of it, Amanda described an experience that was more characteristically consonant. Amanda spent some youthful years in formation in a convent. Weeping with deep feeling, she remembered and spoke of those years:

> *Amanda*: Those years in the convent were the best in my whole life. They just really, really were! And painful as they were . . . I felt so isolated and so lonely . . . I missed my family so much. [long pause] The way the Spirit has moved me. It's really taught me a lot about reflection, meditation, and prayer, creating a space of peace, and of prayer and beauty in [my] home. A space where [I] can sit quietly and think, and be thankful and pray, and just reflect and write, or whatever. There always seems to be a lot of beauty in everything, no matter how ugly it appears at the moment.

Regarding religion and religiosity rejected, and faith and spirituality claimed, I was not surprised that these themes would manifest in the Latinas' description because I know from my own experience that faith, religion, and spiritual practice are important to people of Spanish-Mexican heritage.

Education: Theme 3

In the early days on the northern frontier of Mexico, there was no opportunity for formal education for most families. Even by 1912, when New Mexico gained statehood, "seven school districts in [northern New Mexico's] mountainous Rio Arriba County had no school, and nine-tenths of the schools with teachers met for three months or less. Moreover, the county had no public high school until 1917" (Deutsch, 1987, 65). I

162 Gloria L. Córdova

mention Rio Arriba County in particular because Hispanos largely popu-
lated it at that time. As New Mexico was among the last states to be admitted to the Union, education for its Spanish-Mexican people in remote areas
of the state was seriously lacking. The lack of opportunity that prevailed in
early days has not changed much for many families who live in northern
New Mexico. Several of the women described this disadvantage in their
younger lives, longingly wishing that they might have had the opportunity
for more formal education. Maria Elena recognized her own intelligence as
she expressed her regret that she did not have the opportunity to develop
her education formally beyond high school.

> *Maria Elena*: I always did well in school. I guess I started reading at a very young
> age. I always did well in school. I was pretty smart, and even still I feel [pretty
> smart]. When I was in high school, I wanted to go to college, but not very many
> girls went to college when I was in high school. . . . And nobody ever said, "Go
> to school." [Not] even my counselors! And that's what I really [resent]. You
> know, sometimes when I think about it, I think those counselors were really
> worthless. You know, couldn't they see that [academic talent] in me?

Unlike Maria Elena, I eventually had the opportunity and choice to pursue
advanced education. My father later called me the perpetual student
because I was always in school, most recently completing my Ph.D. at age
sixty-six. Yet the pursuit of higher education can create internal conflict. I
expressed my own experience this way:

> As a woman grows, develops, and matures, and she consciously recognizes that
> her Self has been stifled and silenced. She discovers that her mind and her
> voice are integral to who she is and who she is becoming. The Latina's self
> emerges from many deep layers of old world traditions and beliefs to find her-
> self in new world space, confused with and still bound by the old. She feels
> conflicted and oppressed. A choice she may make for her self-emergence is to
> return to school and higher education. By her choice for education she feels
> liberated yet still conflicted by old traditions versus her new world expecta-
> tions. How does she find her voice? How does she express her voice? (Personal
> Journal Entry, as cited in Córdova, 2004)

Working with the stories of the participants in my study, and reflecting
upon my own opportunities, I came to see myself as a cultural pioneer:

> I was more proud and appreciative of my Spanish heritage than ever before.
> Feelings of low self-esteem were not as prevalent in my life as they had been
> before. I did not feel so victimized. I began the Ph.D. program during this [low-
> esteem/victim] period of my life, after experiencing the fear of job loss when I
> was on the list for a reduction-in-force (RIF). Mother always told me education
> was something no one could ever take from me. The Ph.D. was the epitome of

formal education, something that few Latinas had the privilege of earning. I wanted to increase those numbers by one, determined to model for the Spanish community of men and women that we are capable, we can earn advanced degrees. (Personal Journal Entry, as cited in Córdova, 2004)

This reflection and the other women's comments move us to display the theme of opportunity lost and gained.

Skin Color: Theme 4

The Latinas in this study are descendants of *mestizo* people, those of racially mixed American Indian and European ancestry. Their ancestors were in the land that is now New Mexico four hundred years ago—the very same geographical location, or lived space, where these women reside today. "Regardless of when their ancestors came here [they] are still perceived as women of color, while European and other white immigrants become mainstream Americans as early as the second generation" (Comas-Diaz and Greene, 1994, 4).

Light skin and dark skin remained a central characterization for the Latinas. There has been a clear, though sometimes subtle, discriminatory attitude toward dark-skinned Latinas, which often negatively affects their self-esteem: "Research shows that women who have dark skin, especially with indigenous features, face the worst treatment from society at large" (Zavella, 1991, 78–79). Light-skin sisters experienced an opposite aspect of the discriminatory attitude toward their dark-skin sisters. Though lighter skin gives favored status in families and society, it is painful to be seen as different and privileged. We Norteñas de Nuevo Méjico are descendants of mestizo people, of racially mixed American Indian and European ancestry, and race and racial identification are significant forces in our cultural body:

Internalization of the fundamental dynamic of history and culture always works most insidiously against those who are marked by the signs of skin color, speech, and community. It simultaneously works in favor of those who by virtue of the same signs are unmarked and considered normal. (J. M. Martinez, 2000, 12)

A trio of sisters, Maria Elena and twins Amanda and Sylvia, remembered that their dark-skinned mother used to say resentfully about her sister, "She was so *güera* [fair-skinned] that mother used to take her everywhere." Maria Elena described three of her siblings: "All my older siblings, my three older siblings, are blonde because my father had blonde hair and blue eyes." Maria Elena went on to say, about her two fair-skinned sisters, "Well, see, they could have passed for being white."

The sisters demonstrated an acute awareness of differences in light and dark skin color, as well as resulting differences in treatment in their family.

Maria Elena: I love my brothers to pieces, even my fair-haired brother, because you know he's a good brother. It wasn't his fault that my mother loved him so much. He was very, very blond when he was born.

Amanda: So blond he was white-haired.

Maria Elena: Yeah. His hair was white.

Amanda: So he was more acceptable, more accepted, I think.

Maria Elena: All my older siblings, my three older siblings, are blonde because my father had [all three say together] blonde hair and blue eyes. [Mother] was dark.

Amanda: Probably even darker than us.

Maria Elena: Dark. Yeah, darker than us.

Amanda: Sylvia and I and one of my brothers look a lot like [our mother] as far as complexion goes.

Maria Elena: You know, I think that was a problem with my mother, too, because my mother was dark, and her younger sister, Josie, was very fair. My mom would say that my grandma would take Josie everywhere.

Amanda: That's a very good insight! Our blonde brother never talks about it, does he?

Recognizing the differences in treatment and favoritism toward their fair-skinned and blonde brother, these sisters knew from experience that "a person who is marked, especially by skin color, is always at risk for being stereotyped by racist norms" (J. Martinez, 2000, 81). Whether dark-skinned or fair-skinned, either can occasion oppression. Teresa mentioned her dark-skinned sister's feelings. While there did not appear to be different treatment in the family by reason of skin color, the situation was different beyond their home. Teresa described her feelings of being discriminated against outside her family due to her light skin coloring.

Teresa: We really didn't feel there was that much of a difference in terms that we were treated [at home]. But I know when I went to high school, I remember women classmates saying, "Well, we thought you were a *gringa*." . . . And in college was the first time I ever experienced any kind of discrimination because I was light. Like, I'd show up at the Chicano—that was the first time I ever knew about *Chicano*—I'd show up at the Chicano parties [Teresa laughs here] and I'd get this look like, "Who are you?" You know, for people who didn't want me around, thinking I didn't belong there. It was real hard!

The women's voices tell us of the wound and blessing they experienced with respect to skin color, another expression of the dissonance and consonance resonating through their lives.

Family and Relationships: Theme 5

This theme comprised wounds and blessings of family and relationships relative to several aspects of the women's experiences. The dissonance-consonance is visible through experiences with parental nurturing. Elena expressed a feeling of insignificance in her life, a feeling that she perceives as directly related to her mother's lack of regard for her:

> *Elena*: I always felt like my mom favored the boys much more because, when she was ill, I remember her saying one time that the only thing that saddened her if she died was leaving my little brother. He was three years younger than me. And I thought, "My gosh, doesn't she care if she leaves me?" And I was a little, you know; that just stayed with me. I always felt like I couldn't matter.

By contrast, Martha described a decision of five sisters in her family when her only brother needed a kidney.

> *Martha*: I think that's part of the strength that we have in our family. He needed a kidney, and he was about to go on dialysis, and so I offered him my kidney. And he didn't want to take it, but I said, "Look, you know this is the way we are. If something is broke, let's fix it." And actually then all of my other sisters said, "Yeah, let's do this." And they all volunteered to give him a kidney. And we kind of chose three of us because the others had more responsibilities, like small children . . . so three of us got tested, and I was the closest match. So that is our special bond.

Despite the setbacks of divorce, family-of-origin issues, and poverty, the women described using their experiences as a basis for solving problems in their lives, finding voice, and claiming identity.

Ethnic Identity: Theme 6

The sixth theme of these Latinas' lived experience is ethnic identity and ethnic consciousness development, through the pain and anger of oppression and the blessings and pride in heritage. Their painful personal experiences of oppression also have roots in historical terms. Even early writers who chronicled the southwest (Gregg, 1954; J. J. Webb, 1995; W. P. Webb, 1931) did the early-settler, Spanish-Mexican people no favors in describing what they saw in terms of damaging stereotypes (Acuña, 1998; Garza-Falcon,

1998), which underlie the dissonant experiences of oppression: the dark side of the themes experienced even today.

What was it about our experiences that led us, in varying degrees, to develop our consciousness of ethnic identity? Two aspects of Latinas' ethnic identity are how we identify and the evolving development of our ethnic consciousness. Bernal and Knight (1993) noted that ethnic identity is a particular aspect of the question: "Who am I?" In the deeper meaning of Latinas' stories, including mine, I saw a connection to the Latina feminist traditions of struggle and resistance, for which "history is not only that of victimization but also resistance [to a] colonized mentality" (E. Martinez, 1995, 1020).

Characteristic of Latinas in northern New Mexico, when asked their ethnicity, they will respond across the spectrum from *American, Hispanic, Spanish, Spanish American, Mexican, Mexican American, Latina, Chicana* to *mestiza*. For example, Martha reacted to the term *Mexican American* when she spoke of her own development, in the way she identified earlier and how she now identifies herself. She told of speaking with her husband when she read of an ethnic activist group being formed. He encouraged her to investigate it. He told her that she should not just always deplore the condition of Hispanics but should go do something about it. She told me how she replied to her husband:

> *Martha*: I don't know if I can do this because—Mexican American—boy, I don't really relate to being Mexican American. . . . I know there's something there, you know, that I probably am Mexican American, but we've never identified as such. I [thought], "Mexican American Women's National Association. Is this me?"

Carmela, on the other hand, told me, "I feel it in my heart," when describing herself as a *Mexican*, a *mestiza*. She described the strong reaction to *Mexican* from all her siblings but one brother when she discusses ethnicity with them. Her description clearly depicts the dilemma of ethnic identity among native New Mexicans.

> *Carmela*: You know, I don't think they mean it derogatory or anything, but that's where they [Spanish people who do not identify as Spanish-Mexican] think they came from, Oñate [meaning that they think they are of pure Spanish blood], because we've been told by the Anglo culture that we are that way, and so they believe that. It's in their head. And, I don't think that they have studied who we really are. And I haven't studied it as much as like you or others have studied it, but I feel [it] in my heart.

When asked how I identify, I now can readily reply *Chicana, mestiza,* and *Mexicana*. Years ago, when a close *Tejana* (Texas) friend asked me why I never identified as Mexican-American, I told her I'd never thought about it. Years later, reflecting on her question, I realized that a bias was instilled in me from early childhood about identifying as such. Study of the intersection of gender, race, and class brought the bias to my consciousness. Just as my awareness evolved about who I am, the same is true, to varying degrees, for the other women in this study.

Carmela, for instance, described a "seed" in her mind that awakened her, over time, to consciousness of ethnicity:

> *Carmela*: I have a younger brother who told me about, who put the seed in my mind, about treatment of Hispanics. He is the one who told me about La Raza Unida [a New Mexico political organization that was considered extremist]. He took me to a meeting of the La Raza Unida Party. I was totally shocked. That really opened my eyes. These men were fighting for our rights. This was during the Reyes Lopez Tijerina days [the leader of the La Raza Unida Party]. [I was afraid and thought], "We've got to get out of here. This is too dangerous. Something is going to blow up." They were being violent, but they were being strong. I had never seen anything like it. My brother said, "No, this is our history. We have to fight. We have to help." . . . Ever since then, I've always thanked him for that, because I think that was the seed. It lit the fire [for her raised consciousness, activism, and self-identification as *mestiza*].

While many of the dissonant experiences were attributable to such racial/ethnic discrimination, this attitude made the people hyper-reactive, angry, and even ill. I, for one, recognized that I needed to be able to deal with my anger while standing in testimony to discrimination and oppression. The next section reveals the essence of the phenomena of finding voice and claiming identity, an essential structure connecting all six themes and topics.

DISSONANCE AND CONSONANCE: ESSENCE OF THE PHENOMENON

In determining the essence of the Latinas' experience through these six themes—language, religion, education, skin color, family and relationships, and ethnic identity—and acknowledging the possibility of countless others, I looked for descriptions that brought on feelings and thoughts with reference to the phenomena of finding voice and claiming identity, such as time, space, bodily concerns, materiality, relationship to self, and relation to others. Similarly, I searched for descriptions that vividly illustrated the themes and facilitated the development of a description of these phenomena.

I found that the essence of our experiences is in our genealogy, our ancestral family history. We and our families have always lived in what is now

New Mexico. Although we lived continuously in this same land since the 1600s, as *nativos*, and did not change national or state borders; the political boundaries and even dominant language and culture changed around us. The changed context fueled a lack of deeper understanding of the place of Latinos in a territory increasingly controlled by non-*nativo* newcomers. The stories of the Latinas in the study consistently reflect this history of the hegemony that exists in the United States today. Their stories also indicate how their consciousness developed as they learned to make connections between consciousness and action.

The Latinas' voices were clear about their development. They described painful experiences and spoke of self-destructive anger, giving emotionally touching examples of how self-realization emerged. A particularly insightful moment for Teresa was her realization of how unhealthy her marital situation had been for her before she made the decision to divorce, and how her consciousness was thus embodied:

> *Teresa*: I know one time my sister said—this was when I was operated on for tumors in my uterus— . . . "We're having children and you're creating tumors." [Teresa thought about it five years after her divorce.] I felt like I wanted to create it in that [marriage] situation and it wasn't possible, but I was going to create regardless. So I did. I created fibroids.

It was clear that she had matured greatly from lessons learned in that marriage and divorce, and in her consciousness as a Latina. At another point, Teresa described severe skeletal problems she had had over time, some of them, she thought, due to accidents. She chuckled, "What are my bones trying to tell me? Take more calcium! But aside from that, what else?" Implicit in this embodied learning and change is a growing consciousness development of our Spanish-Mexican, *mestiza* ethnocultural history. Carmela described her awakening awareness and evolving consciousness when she moved from home in New Mexico to work in Washington, DC:

> *Carmela*: [That group of Hispanic friends from Texas] all really awakened my Hispanic heritage in me. It was there, [but] it was like sleep. [I] was asleep. I was going to say it was dead, but I like better the words that it was asleep. It was always there, I think, but it was asleep.

"A mestiza consciousness is far more difficult to grasp for those whose racial and ethnic consciousness is absent, or de-historicized or regarded as something that can be everchangingly shed or adopted at will" (Gonzalez, 1997, 134). The Latinas in the study described moving from lacking awareness about Spanish-Mexican, *mestiza* history to being acutely attuned to their cultural history. They are products of a de-historicized racial and ethnic consciousness. To regain awareness, to be able to take action, required learning and change, with many opportunities to practice.

In our awakening to cultural history and ethnic awareness, I recognized a growing, related political consciousness. Paulo Freire used the Portuguese term *conscientizaçao*, meaning "learning to perceive social, political, and economic contradictions, and to take action against the oppressive elements of reality" (1992, 19). Scholar-activist Gloria Anzaldúa (1987) brought the term into Spanish, *conscientización*, in the same context as Freire's.

Each of the Latinas' life stories involved transformation in personal growth and development. These women came to see themselves differently and behave differently, particularly as they evolved in the consciousness of their ethnic identity as *mestizas*. Each reclaimed pride in her roots as *Latina, Spanish-Mexican, Chicana*, and *mestiza*. They all developed consciousness to speak out and take action against oppression.

NASCENT THEORY: DEVELOPMENT OF *CONSCIENTIZACIÓN*

When considering the insights from my research taken as a whole, I began to see an emerging theory regarding the development of *conscientización*. In carefully reviewing their stories and descriptions, I recognized that there were intervening experiences that forcefully caught the Latinas' attention and raised their awareness. Oppression and discrimination in their lives were described in action, movement, and fluidity, coming out of pain, grief, and distress. In the narratives dwelt the substance of theory.

Latina/Chicana feminists call theory developed from lived experience *theory in the flesh* (Moraga and Anzaldúa, 1983), redefining how theory is written and practiced (Trujillo, 1998). This sense of theory from lived experience—as knowledge implicit in one's history, tradition, and culture—resonated for the Latinas in my study. Saldívar-Hull (2000), for example, advocated looking for theories where you can find them in the non-places of theory. Meaning, understanding, and rationality rise from and are conditioned by our bodily experience (Johnson, 1987).

The research approach (van Manen, 1990) and rich narratives enabled me to build upon the Latinas' lived experience, and my own, through reflection on the work, talking about it, writing about it, and understanding it. I thought about how the Latinas grew and developed in awareness of consciousness. Studying the process brought discovery; theory unfolded as a process of self-authorship, as illustrated in figure 10.1. The ovals in the figure represent the stages in the process, illustrated from bottom to top. The keywords in the figure are italicized in the following discussion.

Development of *Conciencia de la Mestiza*
Reclamation and Reconstruction of Identity

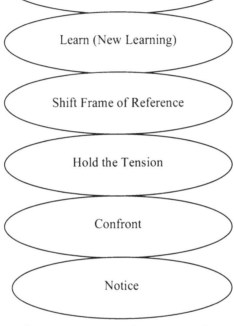

Figure 10.1.   Process of Latina Human Consciousness Development

First, we only *notice* what we notice, because of who we are. We create ourselves by what we choose to notice. We do not notice anything except what confirms who we already think we are. We are self-sealed in our Spanish-Mexican experience, in the world that was significantly influenced by fundamental existentials: our ethnicity, cultural body, spatial geographical location, contextual time in history, and relationships. All of these influences are directly linked to our Spanish-Mexican descendant experience in northern New Mexico and southern Colorado, which is an extension of Spanish-Mexican cultural New Mexico.

Until some intervention, usually life-serious, circumstance or event in our lives occurs to *confront* us, we cannot move outside of our normal processes of self-reference. We experience events that enable us to look at ourselves with real self-awareness, allowing us to live with and *hold the tension* between the dissonant and consonant aspects of our experiences. This results in personal change for us, which comes from a *shift in our frame of reference*. This shift leads us to *learn*, clearly *new learning*. Experiences that were previously considered negative and dissonant can now be experienced as opportunities, that is, positive and consonant experiences. The pain, anger, suffering, anxiety, and chaos of our experiences of internalized oppression can be transcended, with practice and support, through new learning that leads to reclamation and reconstruction of identity. In transcending, we don't leave behind our experiences of oppression. Certainly, we know and remember our history, yet we can still give voice to our experience of pain and pride. We stand *witness* to the world, as we bear witness to the knowledge and memory of our history, and, at the same time, give voice to our experience of pain and pride.

This nascent theory of Latina consciousness development is, I believe, the *conscientizaçao* of which Freire (1992) wrote and the *conscientización* or the *conciencia de la mestiza* of which Anzaldúa (1987) wrote. Many writers have since adopted Anzaldúa's phrase *conciencia de la mestiza*. I use it here as described by Jacqueline M. Martinez (2000): "a description of a successful struggle against the oppressive forces of the dominant culture at the level of the lived body" (84).

To varying degrees, the Latinas who participated in this study reclaimed and reconstructed their lives and their sense of self despite, and in opposition to, the many forms of hegemonic subordination with which they live. The Latinas came to see themselves differently and behave differently by reclaiming and reconstructing their sense of ethnic Spanish-Mexican, *mestiza* self. The new consciousness of self of which Anzaldúa (1987) wrote is the phenomenon of *conscientización*.

In relating the northern New Mexico Latina's consciousness to *conciencia de la mestiza*, I am cognizant of and heeding the strong and valid caution put forth by Jacqueline M. Martinez about entering into a consideration of Anzaldúa's (1987) work:

> Theoretical effort can never be equated to practice. The theoretical effort itself does not entail a one-to-one correspondence between the ideas carried therein and the manifestation of those ideas in the concrete world of human experience. . . . It is important to work against the tendency to simplify, gloss over, or to too quickly valorize the "new consciousness" without committing oneself to the complexity and gut-wrenching struggle out of which theorizing like Anzaldúa's is born. (J. M. Martinez, 2000, 83)

> [Anzaldúa's (1987)] work provides a set of circumstances and practices through which we might create humanizing spaces in our cultural, social, and personal worlds alike. Yet, because it is attentive to the particularities of situation and the possibilities of the lived body, Anzaldúa's work cannot be reduced to a prescription, a set of procedures, or a single perspective that can be copied

as a way to achieve liberating transformations for self and the social world.
(J. M. Martinez, 2000, 84–85)

The consciousness of which I speak is a *critical consciousness*. The northern
New Mexico Latinas, the women in this study, are *mestiza*, "a hybrid, situated between cultures, languages, communities, and histories, with each
foot set on conflicting and incompatible sides" (85).

My study permits self-definition for the participants and makes their
experiences visible. New learning, especially deep learning, is not simple in
life; such learning is gut-wrenching, lived-body learning: "All knowledge is
mediated. One of these mediations is your own flesh which keeps things in
hiding if and until you are ready to get undressed in front of the mirror of
your own being" (Bentz, 2003, 181).

In this work of analysis and interpretation of the narratives, I, too, experienced a personal transformation. I now understand, in my body as well as
in my mind, why consciousness development is imperative for me and
other Latinas. I understand and appreciate what I learned from the phenomenology of the Latinas' lived experience. We carry in our bodies the effects of our cultural, ethnic history. The cultural embodies the terms of its
existence, as does the lived body. Healing is gut-wrenching, lived bodywork.
The kind of knowing that emerges from doing this kind of research is not
something I learned from academic textbooks.

By working with the narratives of the Latinas, and reflecting and writing
about the meaning that the Latinas gave to their actions, I came to recognize the reality of an embodied wisdom in them and myself. This recognition allowed me to write, from the lived experience of the northern New
Mexico Latina's everyday life and lifeworld, a compelling narrative of discovering voice and reclaiming identity. From this embodied wisdom, I was
able to glean new knowledge, build *theory in the flesh*, and contribute to
phenomenological sociology.

A CLOSING NOTE

I have lived both the pain and the pride of my ethnic origin. I am a woman
who was born and raised in a culture of home-family Spanish speakers in
the southwest United States of southern Colorado. By the 1590s, my *an-
tepasados* (ancestors) had traveled *El Camino Real de Tierra Adentro* to the
northern frontier of Mexico, in what is now the state of New Mexico.

My own history brought into focus personal problems that affected my
self-esteem. My life to this point has been a personal journey to develop
self-understanding and self-esteem. I learned to recognize and deal with my
own internalized oppression. I reclaimed pride in my ethnic and cultural

roots. As a result, I weave a different life story for myself now, a more positive story that tells of experiences of more consonance. I also tell the story of the Latina participants:

> I am the storyteller. I give voice to the unspoken stories of simple, strong, phenomenal women. I elicit the telling and sharing of the story of their becoming, their claiming of SELF in all the fullness of beauty, wholeness, and good. I am their *hermana*, the sister of the women of the upper Rio Grande Valley, the northern New Mexico women, the *mestiza*, the wondrously beautiful racial and ethnic mix of Spanish, Mexican, Sephardic Moor, Indian, old-world/new-world woman.
>
> I tell about the strength of women who know their depths because they know how deeply their pain dwelt. I tell of the beauty, the sensitivity, the brilliance, the humanity, the love of these women. They are Latinas who reclaimed and reconstructed their personal identity, were transformed by bringing the unconscious to consciousness, and found their way by laying down their path while walking.
>
> I tell their story to a world enriched by knowing and appreciating their becoming, their story of their process of knowing who they are. I tell their story to their brothers, to their families, to all those who may never know these women, the *prietas*, the *güeras*, the *coyotas*, the *Chicana*, the *mestiza*, the *Mexicana—las mujeres de la tierra del sol*—the women of the land of the sun.

REFERENCES

Acuña, Roldolfo F. (1998) *Occupied America: A History of Chicanos* (fourth ed.). New York: Longman.

Anzaldúa, Gloria. (1987) *Borderlands/La Frontera: The New Mestiza*. San Francisco: Aunt Lute.

Aquino, Maria P., Daisy L. Machado, and Jeanette Rodriguez (Eds.). (2002) *A Reader in Latina Feminist Theology: Religion and Justice*. Austin: University of Texas Press.

Bentz, Valerie (2003) The Body's Memory, the Body's Wisdom. In Matti Itkonen and Gary Backhaus (Eds.), *Lived Images: Mediations in Experience, Life-World and I-Hood* (158–84). Finland: Jyvaskyla University Press.

Bernal, Martha E., and George P. Knight (Eds.). (1993) *Ethnic Identity: Formation and Transmission Among Hispanics and Other Minorities*. Albany: State University of New York Press.

Briggs, Charles L. (1999) *Learning How to Ask: A Sociolinguistic Appraisal of the Role of the Interview in Social Science Research* (vol. 1). New York: Cambridge University Press.

Comas-Diaz, Lillian, and Beverly Greene (Eds.). (1994) *Women of Color: Integrating Ethnic and Gender Identities in Psychotherapy*. New York: Guilford Press.

Córdova, Gloria L. (2004) *The Lived Experience of Norteñas de Nuevo Méjico: Finding Voice and Reclaiming Identity*. Unpublished Ph.D. Dissertation. Santa Barbara, CA: Fielding Graduate Institute.

de la Torre, Adela, and Beatriz M. Pesquera (Eds.). (1993) *Building with Our Hands: New Directions in Chicana Studies*. Berkeley: University of California Press.

Deutsch, Sarah. (1987) *No Separate Refuge: Culture, Class, and Gender on an Anglo-Hispanic Frontier in the American Southwest, 1880–1940*. New York: Oxford University Press.

Ebright, Malcolm. (1994) *Land Grants and Lawsuits in Northern New Mexico*. Albuquerque: University of New Mexico Press.

Esquibel, José A. (1998) Founding Mothers of New Mexico: The Perez de Bustillo Women. *El Farolito, 1*(2), 15–18.

Esquibel, José A., and Douglas Preston. (1998) *The Royal Road: El Camino Real from Mexico City to Santa Fe*. Albuquerque: University of New Mexico Press.

Freire, Paulo. (1992) *Pedagogy of the Oppressed*. New York: Continuum.

Garza-Falcon, Leticia M. (1998) *Gente Decente: A Borderlands Response to the Rhetoric of Dominance*. Austin: University of Texas Press.

González, Deena J. (1997) Chicana Identity Matters. *Aztlan, 22*(2), 123–38.

—— (1999) *Refusing the Favor: The Spanish-Mexican Women of Santa Fe, 1820–1880*. New York: Oxford University Press.

Gregg, Josiah. (1954) *Commerce of the Prairies* (vol. 17). Norman: University of Oklahoma Press.

Johnson, Mark. (1987) *The Body in the Mind: The Bodily Basis of Meaning, Imagination, and Reason*. Chicago: University of Chicago Press.

Martinez, Elizabeth. (1995) In Pursuit of Latina Liberation. *Signs, 20*(4), 1019–28.

Martinez, Jacqueline M. (2000) *Phenomenology of Chicana Experience and Identity: Communication and Transformation in Praxis*. Lanham, MD: Rowman & Littlefield.

Moraga, Cherrie, and Gloria Anzaldúa (Eds.). (1983) *This Bridge Called My Back: Writings by Radical Women of Color* (second ed.). New York: Kitchen Table/Women of Color Press.

Saldívar-Hull, Sonia. (2000) *Feminism on the Border: Chicana Gender Politics and Literature*. Berkeley: University of California Press.

Trujillo, Carla (Ed.). (1998) *Living Chicana Theory*. Berkeley: University of California Press.

van Manen, Max. (1990) *Researching Lived Experience: Human Science for an Action Sensitive Pedagogy*. London, Ontario, Canada: State University of New York Press.

Webb, James J. (1995) *Adventures in the Santa Fe Trade, 1844–1847* (Bison Book ed.). Lincoln: University of Nebraska Press.

Webb, Walter P. (1931) *The Great Plains*. New York: Ginn.

Zavella, Patricia (1991) Reflections on Diversity Among Chicanas. *Frontiers—A Journal of Women's Studies, 12*(2), 73–85.

11

A Breath of Fresh Air

Phenomenological Sociology and Tai Chi

Marc J. LaFountain

It is always difficult to determine how shallow your breath is until you breathe deeply. It is difficult to say how constricted, tight, and drawn in you become when in crisis until you flow openly into your surrounding spaces. It is difficult to tell how unbalanced and uncollected you are until the alignment that you assume you have with your self and body is revealed to be an awkward heaviness that masks as a kind of lightness that is actually flimsy and easily uprooted.

I begin with the 2000 winter solstice. The winter solstice marks the time when the sun is the farthest from the equator, hence the short spell of light on the shortest and darkest day of the year. Envisioned as an ecliptic, which traces the sun's path around the earth, it is said that the winter solstice is the highest point in that movement, where the sun seems to stand still for a moment.

The 2000 winter solstice was the date that the legal papers terminating my dozen-year-old marriage were finalized and signed. The trek to the courthouse was made in heavy gray light, cold winds, intermittent sleet, and snow showers. It was the shortest, darkest day of the year, the temperatures were chilling, and I was in shock of what I had not asked for or expected. I was at the limit, far from myself, just doing what I needed to do to take care of only the most necessary and pressing details of daily living. My breath was short and superficial. Yet I felt keenly alive and paradoxically open in those moments that dragged me along.

DISRUPTION AS AN OPENING

The story of the relationship's unraveling is not necessary to recount here. Having informed me of her departure in mid-October, she left in the darkness of Halloween. I couldn't fathom the cold or gloom, the symbolism of the Halloween exit and the final ending on the shortest, darkest day. I didn't ask, nor did it really matter then, but somehow a story seemed imminent. A narrative began forming. Within days of Thanksgiving, I joined a small tai chi class. For years, I had wanted to learn tai chi, and earlier in the year I had heard glowing reports of an instructor newly moved to my community. My earliest interest in martial arts started during my college freshman days. I had enrolled to study judo. My instructor was a frail man more than three times my age. I found that I could not deal with the throws, falls, and bone locks. Later, I entertained karate, but abandoned the idea after considering the stresses on a surgically repaired knee. When I was most uprooted and estranged from the connection I already was to myself, tai chi made sense.

My teacher's strategy was for us to learn first the mechanics of the long form of the yang style of tai chi. When he demonstrated the entire form, with all its postures and motions, I couldn't imagine how I could learn all of that. He said he would introduce other crucial elements, particularly breathing, push hands, and martial applications, as we learned the basic form. It didn't register, then, how important breathing is to moving, rootedness, adhering, and releasing. We were instructed to read Lowenthal's (1993) *There are No Secrets*, about Master Cheng Man-ch'ing's rendition of tai chi. I was intrigued by Master Cheng's smile; I wanted to know what he knew.

I was struck by how awkward I felt as I tried to learn the most elementary aspects of reconfiguring my posture, movement, and balance. As it dawned on me that I was unlearning as well as learning, I realized that the shock of the unfamiliar that I was experiencing was similar to what I ask of my students in my phenomenological sociology course, "The Sociology of Everyday Life." I also noted the coincidence of the shock of my solstice divorce and what is necessary to practice phenomenology as a prelude to its application in sociology. For phenomenology begins with shock and crisis. What this shock facilitates can be as life-altering as events such as divorces or learning new ways of moving.

INTENTIONALLY ALTERING THE TAKEN FOR GRANTED

Phenomenology requires that we separate ourselves from what we know, or temporarily suspend what we know in order to grasp this knowing as it comes to be. Letting go of the natural attitude—the taken-for-granted, trusted, and forgotten assumptions guiding everyday life—is shocking and disorienting. Harold Garfinkel's *breaching* experiments not only opened students' eyes to a world of tacit expectations, but also shocked them as they tried to suspend those very same assumptions in order to complete the experiments (1967). Without some breach of what we take for granted, we forget how much the taken for granted infuses our every thought, movement, and breath.

To prepare my students for doing phenomenological reflection, they complete the *McGrane experiment*. This experiment is described in Bernard McGrane's *The Un-TV and the 10 MPH Car*. In this Zen-inspired approach to doing sociology, McGrane warns, in the first chapter, that studying sociology can be "harmful to your ego" because it treats sociology as a way of being and, once begun, it is difficult to reverse (1994, 9). Students learn what this means by completing the book's first exercise, "Unoccupied, Unemployed." The instructions are to select a place where people are interacting; be there for ten minutes; do nothing—be unoccupied and unemployed; see what you see; and, once the exercise is completed, write a description of what you perceived and felt.

This exercise is done in the first week or two of the semester. Simultaneously, students are introduced to phenomenological sociology as a variant of qualitative sociology. The McGrane exercise serves two purposes. It acquaints students with the Zen notion of *beginner's mind*, which, in many ways, is related to what one does when *bracketing* one's interpretive framework.[1] Both operations clear the mind of its preconceptions, so as to perceive in a fresh and open manner, as if for the first time. The exercise also shocks individuals, in that it confronts them with how much they take for granted. Acknowledging the depth and subtlety of what is assumed grounds the beginner's mind and bracketing in immediate experience.

Parallel to the McGrane experiment, and as an introduction to phenomenology itself, the students read David Rehorick's (1986) "Shaking the Foundations of Lifeworld: A Phenomenological Account of an Earthquake Experience" and S. Kay Toombs's (2001) "Reflections on Bodily Change: The Lived Experience of Disability." They are instructed to select several phenomenologically relevant concepts and ideas from the readings and lectures and apply them to their descriptions of their McGrane experience. Doing this introduces Alfred Schutz's crucial distinction between first and second order constructs. *First-order constructs*, individuals' interpretations, and narratives of their lived experiences, are the data that phenomenological sociologists process via their own conceptually laden *second-order constructs*: for example, prethematic meaning, the lived body, or transcendence. Later, the students learn about *intercorporeal perception* and are able to include it as part of their data.

As students delve into the subtle facets of moment-to-moment, everyday experiences, they discover a new awareness. They become sensitive to the experiences of those who lived through the earthquake, as they struggled to place its uncanny irruption in their lifeworlds into a familiar context. Likewise, via Toombs's everyday struggles with multiple sclerosis, they become attentive to life with an unpredictable body. Becoming aware of these ordeals leads to an appreciation of understanding the (social) world as others experience it. On a much deeper level, one becomes sensitive to the operations of the mind, the body, and their intricate interconnections as the grounds or means by which we know our selves and others.

In addition to the examples by Rehorick and Toombs, Arthur Frank's essay on illness and storytelling highlights the significance of how we grapple with the shock of the unfamiliar through storytelling. Frank's study of cancer patients and others with serious illnesses focuses not so much on their experience of illness itself—its disruptions and crises—but on how individuals reestablish their identities and relations with others. Frank notes that, when one's life is radically dislocated by illness, part of the shock is that one enters a private province that others have difficulty reaching or understanding, except by falling back on typified and clichéd recipes about what the sick or dying are experiencing or what it means. The *province of meaning* that the seriously ill inhabit can only be opened to others through the stories that the ill tell (2001, 233). These stories create bridges from their lived experience to that of others. Storytelling creates the conditions for new ways for the ill to understand themselves, for finding new ways to help others understand them, and for the creation of *moral subjects*. Moral subjects are those attentive to what they value in their own and others' lives.

> Storytelling is a natural reaction to the shock after which the natural attitude no longer unifies and renders coherent the world. It is a natural reaction to consciousness having to deal with its fundamental anxiety no longer being bracketed but becoming thematic. (242–43)

Frank's mention of the *fundamental anxiety* underlies a crucial element of taken-for-granted, everyday life: death as the horizon against which or in relation to which "I" lives its daily life. What becomes thematic in any disruption is crisis and loss. In many cases, the sense of crisis is mild or little more than an inconvenience or distraction. Here, death is metaphoric—an end to what is possible. As they become more profound and poignant, loss and crisis literally become the being-there of death. Schutz observes, of the fundamental anxiety:

> It is the primordial anticipation from which all others originate. From the fundamental anxiety spring the many interrelated systems of hopes and fears, which incite man within the natural attitude to attempt the mastery of the

world, to overcome obstacles, to draft projects, and to realize them. (1971, 228)

When the fundamental anxiety becomes thematic, it moves from its position of silent backdrop to a haunting presence. For some, whose sense of crisis is relentless, for example, the chronically ill, the disabled, those whose grief or suffering is unrequited, "shock becomes the *continuing* and perpetually elaborating consciousness of one's difference" (Frank, 2001, 235). Whether mild, profound, or perpetually elaborating, shock, and the specter of death that travels with it, must somehow be integrated into one's natural attitude. Such an integration evokes the notion of transcendence.

TRANSCENDENCE, COHERENCE, AND OPENING

Because the embodied "I" inhabits the space and time of here and now, and because the embodied "I" must move from one here and now to another, and so on, in order to dominate and bring the world within its reach so it can accomplish its projects, transcendence is essential. *Transcendence* refers to moving from one here and now to another, whether that movement is in physical or virtual space, or memory, or cognitive, emotional, or spiritual space. To transcend is to go beyond what is beyond. Ideally, transcendence is forward moving, unproblematic, progressive, as if an evolution toward something pragmatically, positively, and coherently meaningful. But meaningfulness can also be expressed as inhibited, interrupted, incomplete, ambiguous, deferred, and/or inestimable.

To transcend a particular here and now is also to move beyond the raw, immediate experience and sense, or even thematic meaning, of a particular lived reality, toward another here and now that is different. To be unable to emerge from the immediacy of that one experiential moment is to be laden with or mired in immanence, a kind of being stuck. Immanence and transcendence, each in its own way, are highly significant. Their dialectical, mutually elaborating relations assure that time and space, and the very movement of subjectivity and intersubjectivity, are experienced as emergence. But therein lies the rub.

Alfred Schutz and Thomas Luckmann's essay, "The Boundaries of Experience and the Boundary Crossings," effectively captures the problems and significance of transcendence (1989). They identify *little, medium,* and *great* transcendencies, and their relation to the wide-awake, *paramount reality* of everyday life. *Little transcendencies* deal with those boundaries of the world that are easily crossable, within my reach. They deal with movement in space and time, such as going from the first floor, where I teach, to my office on the second floor, where my lunch awaits me; remembering in the grocery store, later in the afternoon, the items that I identified in the morning as necessary for my evening meal; and recollecting, when I drove by the hardware store and saw the rakes and hoes, that I forgot to sign up for my gardening class. With little transcendencies, I move around in physical space, back and forth in the present, and between the past, present, and future, as I complete mundane projects each day. I use indicators and marks as media to ease these transitions, where *indicators* are things in the world that call my attention to things that are relevant, such as the rake at the hardware store, and *marks* are intentional indicators that I make for myself, such as notes, dates on calendars, or shoes that I place near my car keys to remember to have them repaired. I readily shift zones of relevance and, as I complete my projects, the fundamental anxiety is silently at bay.

Medium transcendencies are concerned with intersubjectivity. They deal with those boundaries that separate one consciousness from another, yet which can be crossed. For Schutz and Luckmann, these are most significant, because they bear on the social world and, without their successful accomplishment, social reality collapses into a heap of private subjectivities that miscommunicate or pass each other unknowingly. Face to face with each other in direct we-relations, we see one another's bodies and gestures and, via appresentation, we assume the other has a mind or consciousness like our own. Schutz and Luckmann observe that a *dual mediacy*, comprising typifications and what we sense of the other's immediately given body, makes it possible for us to know the other. This knowledge, drawing on a stock of typifications, is constructed via acts of reflection. The medium for crossing the boundary to the other Schutz calls *signs*, which are similar to *symbols* for a symbolic interactionist. They are interpretations of verbal and nonverbal gestures that bring news about and send information to the other. When reciprocally shared, the meanings constituted here form a language. Signs are marks specifically meant for the other. Intersubjectivity, for Schutz, is thus accomplished via the mind's acts of reflection. For Schutz, meaning is only thematic when it is produced retroflectively; that is, one must *step back* from immediate experience in order to reflect and grasp its significance.

Maurice Merleau-Ponty, on the other hand, articulates intersubjectivity in its prereflective or prethematic state as intercorporeality, a primitive or prototypical intersubjectivity because it provides a sense, or unthematized meaning, prior to acts of reflection (1945/1962). Merleau-Ponty provides the crucial element of the embodiment of the "I" that Schutz tends to pass over. Whether focusing on intersubjectivity or intercorporeality, medium transcendencies refer to how we experientially connect with one another. The dialectic of prereflective/reflective awareness, like the dialectic of immanence/transcendence, makes sociality possible.

Through *great transcendencies*, we are able to move back and forth between different realities or finite provinces of meaning. For Schutz, the wide-awake domain of practical activity is *the paramount reality*. Other realities are dreams, sleep, daydreams, fantasy, science, art, ecstatic states, and death. Each province of meaning has its own unique tensions of consciousness and meanings. It is important to be able to import those meanings into the paramount reality, to understand how typical knowledge, developed in the paramount reality, is crucial for making sense of meanings from those other provinces (see Berger and Luckmann's 1966/1967 discussion of the *symbolic universe*), and, further, to consider how meanings from everyday life shape or color what is experienced in other realities. Schutz notes that *symbols* are the media used to cross the boundaries between the paramount and other of the multiple realities.

In all three of the transcendencies, there is the problem that something transcends or is beyond me, and the possibility that I can transcend what transcends me. While it can be assumed that transcendence occurs unproblematically, numerous situations confront us with obstinate boundaries. Rehorick, for instance, discusses the *effortful possibilizing* and reliance on *shields* necessary to create a sense of continuity and closure between one's embodied self and the surroundings it inhabits (1986). Toombs describes her disability as a disruption of the unified body/world system that arose from the disruption of the body as an orientational and intentional locus in the system (2001). The taken-for-granted *I can do it again* of this locus was something upon which she could not rely. Patricia Lengermann and Jill Niebrugge (1995) and Iris Young (1990) describe, from a feminist standpoint, how gender can facilitate or inhibit transcendence. Lengermann and Niebrugge observed how patriarchal domination distorts the we-relation described by Schutz, resulting in experience of *instrumental invisibility* and *instrumental intimacy*. Here, the reciprocity of the *we* becomes one-sided, as the subjectivity of the dominated is eclipsed. Young explores feminine body comportment, motility, and spatiality, and describes in detail how women in sexist society are *handicapped* because of how they learn to move in and utilize space. She argues that the gendered body of the woman contends with "ambiguous transcendence, inhibited intentionality, and discontinuous unity" (1990, 147).

MENTAL AND EMBODIED REFLECTION

The two major traditions within phenomenological sociology referred to above approach reflection differently: Schutz cognitively and Merleau-Ponty from the body. In Schutz's approach, meaning arises primarily via acts of mentalistic and immediate reflection. Prereflective experience is pregnant but mute about what things mean. Merleau-Ponty argues that the prereflective experience is, in fact, a kind of corporeal reflection on meanings that are already emerging in immediate experience. Though ambiguous and in need of the further articulation that time and cognitive reflection provide, prereflective experience is rich with significance. The difference between Schutz and Merleau-Ponty's approaches is captured succinctly in James Ostrow's (1990) *Social Sensitivity* (for a review, see LaFountain, 1992).

I have discovered that, pedagogically, those unfamiliar with phenomenological sociology are better able to grasp these two related, yet different, approaches if Schutz's reflective model is presented prior to Merleau-Ponty. Intuitively and logically, it would make sense that the prereflective's antedating of the reflective would dictate the order of presentation. Intellectually and experientially, however, students report that is not the case. A possible reason for the difficulty in grasping prereflective experience is that it is more immediate, ambiguous, and primordial. Of course, as Ostrow suggests, there are ideological reasons embedded in the dual histories of philosophy and sociology, one instance being that only in the last quarter of the twentieth century did sociology take seriously the issues of embodiment and emotion.

That students grasp themes related to feeling and embodiment more readily after cognitive reflection was also something I discovered in learning tai chi. Tai chi only begins to be clear when the practitioner begins to get a sense of the intrinsic energy (the *chi*) that animates all living things and their relations. Essential to the motility of this energy is breathing, its comings and goings, on which tai chi's postures and movements are predicated. When deep breathing is synchronized with the flow of postures, the subtle power and evasiveness of tai chi are revealed.

But the breathing that tai chi focuses upon is not typical breathing, which is relatively shallow and centered in the chest. With such breathing, the lungs do not expand to capacity, and when they do, the upper chest, above the solar plexus, expands. In deep breathing, the breath sinks into the lower abdomen, below the stomach and navel, where tai chi masters suggest that *chi energy* is stored. The sinking of the breath is crucial to the rooting of the body in its environment, which enhances its adherence, flexibility, balance, and power.

It is difficult to synchronize tai chi postures and movements with deep breathing. Initially, the practitioner experiences a cognitive shock, because the forms being learned require considerable concentration so that the typical, old ways of standing, stepping, and moving can be relearned. The corporeal style and the paths of the habitual body provide a resistance that must be attended to until new habits are embodied. Such cognitive work cannot initially incorporate the subtly complex relations between motility and spatiality. When deep breathing is finally intentionally incorporated into postures and movements, concentration is again required. Occasionally, the new student will stumble upon the seemingly natural ways that certain movements require breathing. But in the choreography of multiple postures and movements, the synchronization of movement and breath is accomplished in tandem with attention to obstacles or opponents in one's environment (obstacles or opponents might be physical, emotional, mental, or spiritual). Only then does one begin to fully grasp tai chi. Many arduous years of practice, reflection, and meditation must pass before one can consider approaching mastery.

Tai chi teaches that it is not only the self, or "I," that organizes experience, but rather temporality, which necessarily implies spatiality in which dynamic life energy (chi) unfolds. Merleau-Ponty captures this sense beautifully:

> I am a field, an experience. One day, once and for all, something was set in motion which, even during sleep, can no longer cease to see or not to see, to feel or not to feel, to suffer or be happy, to think or rest from thinking, in a word 'to have it out' with the world. There then arose . . . a fresh *possibility of situations*. . . . I am . . . one single temporality which is engaged, from birth, in making itself progressively explicit. (1945/1962, 406–7)

The distinguishing feature of embodied consciousness is that consciousness "is in the first place not a matter of 'I think that' but of 'I can'" (Merleau-Ponty, 1945/1962, 137). For Merleau-Ponty, the "I can" is fundamentally embedded in movement and space. The "I can" yields a sense of the world within my reach and is always, necessarily, at work in dealing with any of the boundaries and their crossings noted above, in the discussion of little, medium, and great transcendencies. Because the body inhabits space and time, its basic relation to the world is one of being in the world rather than knowing the world.

At this point, we can return to several matters raised above: students' difficulty in grasping prereflective experience, the difficulty associated with grasping tai chi, and the disruption necessarily associated with new learning, which made me a student learning anew. Students seem to grasp the mentalistically oriented approach of Schutz more readily than the corporeally committed approach of Merleau-Ponty because understanding reflective experience is a matter of knowing and understanding prereflective experience: that is, of being and, only then, knowing. Habituation occurs in both, and when that sediment is disturbed or dislodged, one first falls back on typical recipes for comprehending what has occurred (e.g., Rehorick's effortful possibilizing). The disruption of mental or cognitive sediment can affect one deeply because what one knows goes away or is ineffective. When the disruption of the habitual occurs at the prereflective, corporeal level, the consequences affect one's being: not what one knows, but what one is.

Here the oft-noted ambiguity of Merleau-Ponty's phenomenology of the body becomes salient. Ambiguity refers not to an inadequate method, but rather to an encounter with what it is about us that is opaque, enigmatic, elusive, and mysterious. Prereflective consciousness is the medium in which reflective consciousness comes to life. One must be careful, here, not to take this as a reiteration of the mind/body dualism that phenomenology rejects, for knowing and being are ineluctably intertwined. To a certain degree, one is what one knows, but, even when one does not know, one is. Therein lies the radicality of that which is already always there that is unreflected upon when reflection concerns itself with knowing objects and things.

When students perform the McGrane exercise (of being unoccupied, un-employed), they encounter not just that they held typifications about others, themselves, and the socially constructed meanings of everyday life. They also happen upon their lived bodies as the medium for having a world of everyday life. They discover the significance of Merleau-Ponty's notion that not only do I have a body, but I also *am* my body. Their socially constructed stocks of knowledge are disrupted, which is unsettling, but even more, they report disruptions occurring beyond or behind what thought can express. They report this discomfort in terms of bodily states: emotions, feelings, moods, and senses. Their discomforted corporeal styles are themselves ex-pressions of their encounters with a plurality of layers of meaning built upon lived experience that has now come into view.

Initially, their descriptions of their shock focus on what they took for granted about what they thought. Inevitably, though, they become more focused on the very ways they were attuned to their situations. And ini-tially, it made pedagogical sense to explore their typified knowledge via Schutz's approach. The experiment, however, proved to be invaluable for that point later in the semester where it is necessary to explore issues of the body, particularly the relationship between intersubjectivity and in-tercorporeality. Over the years, students have playfully referred to the Mc-Grane experiment as *the migraine experiment*. Yet they also acknowledge how what it taught them made understanding Merleau-Ponty and Os-trow's insights easier.

Likewise, as I moved through the days and months surrounding the di-vorce, it was my experiences of the social sensitivities of my lived body that were most poignant. In a way, it was as though the body had just irrupted into my presence, announcing itself as if it had a mind of its own. The var-ious feelings, emotions, and senses I experienced as crises were expressions of the degree to which my habitual body had been disrupted. Experiences such as being vulnerable, raw, uneasy, of feeling small, as if withered or withdrawn, expressed the ways in which I was out of sorts with the world that I habitually inhabited. I sensed and felt at my core that the world was no longer familiar, or home: that place where familiarity permits the body and the world to disappear. Drew Leder notes that it is in illness, pain, or suffering that the body *dys-appears*. By this he means that the taken-for-granted body disappears only to dys-appear (dysfunctional appearing) when it is disrupted (1990).

But it was not just my sense of my self and body that was dys-appearing, for the disruption also colored my interactions with others. I did not feel comfortable around others. I experienced this not just in terms of typical intersubjective relations; I experienced it intercorporeally. I felt out of touch with others, as if disconnected, or connected awkwardly, at a level that precedes the kinds of connections that occur in talking or doing things together. The ordinary ease with which I would move in and out of the presence of others, as if a dance I knew by heart, had become a halting, disjointed movement that was unchoreographed, or choreographed badly by someone with no sense of rhythm, coordination, or balance. I did not stay off by myself because of these feelings; these feelings were an expression of that very dys-appearing connectedness.

My awkwardness with others operated as an expression of a social sensitivity that no longer worked to make sense of situations.[2] Even though it no longer worked, it was the stock or reserve on which I drew and, more importantly, as prereflective experience, it occurred simultaneously, such that it was already at work committing or producing me before I could do anything about it. That would change with time, of course, but the significance of this primordial level of signification was that I was already expressing a broken or poorly aligned connection with my world.

FROM SHOCK TO FLOW

In a condition that is not in some way disrupted by a shock or some sort of intentional alteration of consciousness, prethematic social sensitivity disappears. It appears in disruption, toiling in silence behind the scenes. Social sensitivity is not a taken-for-granted *stock of knowledge*, in Schutz's terms, but a prereflective readiness for situations that is available for reflective interpretation. Prereflective experience is complicit with the world, a kind of unconscious reflection, unlike the mentalistic reflection advocated by Schutz. Mentalistic reflection takes for granted this more primitive reflection, or sensitivity. The medium of this sensitivity is corporeality—the lived body—which itself is a "thickness of sensitivity that not only 'orients to' or 'intends' the world, but also has its qualities and intensities, undergoes and embodies them, each moment thereby 'driven into time like a wedge'" (Ostrow, 1990, 31).

When both embodied sensitivity and stocks of reflective interpretation are disrupted, what is disturbed is our very adhesion to or cohesion with the world. By in-habiting the world, we are always connected to it prior to objective knowledge of that cohesion. When this is disrupted, our whole way of knowing and being must be reconstructed. Without such revitalization, disruption sets in minimally as chronic stress and faulty attentiveness, which can warp health, well-being, and relationships. Strangely enough, once new recipes for thinking and being are established, a sense of normalcy and typicality returns, and our actions show "all the marks of habituality, automatism, and half-consciousness" (Schutz, 1964c, 101).

Although habituality, automatism, and half-consciousness have the ring of an undesirable inattentiveness or obliviousness, what is at stake in their not being in place is our ability to flow. According to Charlotte Bloch, mainstream social science has paid little attention to the experience of flow (2000). Doing so, particularly in the context discussed here, dilates our understanding of the habituality, automatism, and half-consciousness to which Schutz refers. Arguably, one could consider Schutz's observation to have a negative connotation. Yet flow is crucial for transcendence from one here and now to another, across the little, medium, and great transcendencies. While transcendence deals with boundary crossings per se, flow can be considered a quality or intensity that denotes optimal transcendence.

Flow suggests a departure from, or a disruption of, mundane reality that is positive and uplifting while, at the same time, it is an intense attentiveness to, and immersion in, a multiplicity of ways of inhabiting the space and time of that very mundane reality. The ecstatic nature of flow experiences creates an uplifting mood, where individuals are more sensitively tuned to their surroundings. Flow, of course, cannot always be maintained continuously over time, but the ability to experience it regularly, as part of one's life, is an expression of vitality and a positive attunement to one's becoming. Conversely, focused attentiveness itself can increase the incidence of flow experiences. This flow is, for students of phenomenology and tai chi alike, an experience of the immediacy that animates life.

THE RECIPROCITY OF TEACHING AND LEARNING

Little did I realize, when I began my study of tai chi, that the unfolding of my life at that time paralleled, in an uncanny way, the progression of ideas that I had built into my syllabus for examining everyday life.[3] At the time that I began learning tai chi, I only knew that I finally had the opportunity to do something that I had long wanted to do. Soon, I discovered that what I was experiencing mimicked the course's conceptual framework. The course's substantive and thematic program itself followed the phenomenological approach to everyday life: that is, to suspend the taken for granted, to recognize the difference between the natural attitude and phenomenological attentiveness to the constitution of mindful, embodied meaning, and to apply what was learned from that difference to re-searching and narrating everyday life. In taking up tai chi, I became poignantly aware of my unbalanced world, my efforts to learn new ways of inhabiting the world, and understanding the power of stories and new narratives to effect that realignment.

Events in my life had assured that I suspended what Schutz refers to as the epoche of everyday life. I could no longer suspend doubt that things were other than what they appeared to be. Everything was different. My capacity to assume, to transcend, to flow and experience a coherent world had been dismantled. I had set up the course, via the McGrane exercise and the readings, to provide a glimpse of what comes to view when the trusted world is impaired or sundered. I had also set up the flow of ideas to move through Schutz's study of reflective consciousness and into Merleau-Ponty's in order to highlight the embodied mind. I had hoped to show that trust, disruption and loss, transcendence, and healing are an ongoing, everyday dynamic. I was poignantly living through what I was teaching.

As I learned tai chi, I was initially preoccupied with a mental understanding of the form and mechanics of its movements and postures. As I learned, the transition to a focus on embodying the form became predominant. My instructor's discussions of tai chi as an internal art slowly became more apparent, for tai chi is not simply a martial art or a new age health routine. It is a way of being, of living, practiced and lived on the highway, in the hardware store, in the kitchen, in the garden, and in all interactions with one's self and others. I discovered for myself what I had reiterated countless times to my own students: One must practice incessantly to maintain a sense of the importance of the relationship between disruption and attentiveness. With tai chi, like the Tao, there is never completion, so the practitioner can never settle for the assumption that the form has been learned and mastery has occurred. Behind and beyond the form always lay surprise, wonder, mystery, and the unknown. Everyday life, which itself is an artful production, is essentially incomplete.

The more I learned about tai chi, the richer my practice of phenomenological sociology became, particularly in the classroom. Teaching phenomenological sociology always requires instruction about how to see the world from another's point of view. What is often lost in this enterprise, however, are the little things that are subtle and seemingly insignificant. For instance, very early in the semester, when students perform the McGrane experiment, class discussions reveal how difficult most find it to do. Many note that they became nervous, insecure, aware of their bodies and the ambient light, sounds, and smells of their environment. Inevitably, several always mention that they had to take deep breaths to calm themselves. At that point, I ask them all to stand and take a deep breath. Analyzing this deep breath, most discovered that a deep breath simply means expanding the lungs so as to puff up the chest. Except for several athletes, dancers, meditation practitioners, singers, and women who had given birth, most do not know how to breathe deeply. As noted above, most think that it means using only the part of the chest above the solar plexus, as if the lower abdomen were irrelevant. I discuss with them how, in the practice of tai chi, breath has physical and spiritual significance. Having done this and offering a demonstration of correct deep breathing, they acknowledge the significant difference between puffing up and proper deep breathing. Many who become interested pursue their practice of deep breathing and report an increased ability to gather, calm, and attune themselves to situations.

Another instance occurred in discussing Young's essay, "Throwing Like a Girl," on the enculturation of gendered embodiment (1990). Students were confident that they knew to what Young's analysis referred. They invoked certain typical images of girls throwing awkwardly, as if such awkwardness were inherent in being a female. Of course, they noted that many women, especially now, are athletic and do not throw like girls. To deepen their appreciation, I asked how many of them were naturally right- or left-handed. I then asked them to stand and make a throwing motion with their non-natural hand. Typically, this throwing motion is somewhat clumsy and unpracticed (except for the ambidextrous). This brings into focus that there is a complex interaction between how they naturally enter the world and how they have been enculturated. Here, they noticed, as Young observes, that comportment and motility involve spatiality (151). With their dominant hands, they found that the throwing motion is accompanied by a fluid way in which they move into and inhabit the surrounding space, whereas throwing with the non-dominant hand uses less space, hence less motility and less balanced coordination.

I then demonstrated several simple tai chi movements, for example, *grasp sparrow's tail*, *roll back*, and *brush knee, twist step*. I asked them to perform the movements. Once they had done this several times, I then demonstrated how to breathe in and out during the motions. When they coordinated breathing with the motions, they were amazed that they didn't pay attention to this relationship, and that it was more flowing and *natural*.

The reciprocities between practicing phenomenology and tai chi also deepened my appreciation of Frank's important discussion of the *formation of a moral subject*. The *moral subject* is one who asks and answers two fundamental questions: "What do I value in my own life?" and "How do I and others express to each other what we value about each other?" (2001, 242). Frank notes that we typically respond to these questions tacitly, but shocks make storytelling and narrating our experiences and our relations to others essential for forming our own self-understanding and communities of meaning. We cannot effectively formulate alone how we respond to life's demands because we are caught up in the lives of others. We need to know how to respond to them and what we need of them. An attuned moral subject does not necessarily rely on being shocked to voice these interests.

Phenomenology and tai chi can increase our appreciation that we are: (a) inseparable from the world we inhabit, (b) both passively and actively in the world (yin and yang), (c) becoming in space and time, (d) experiencing transcendence, and (e) responsible for ourselves and others. We can use narratives to reflect on the meaning of our experiences as embodied consciousness. Both phenomenology and tai chi tune our attentiveness to what is available in mental reflection and what is available to us via the lived body as a medium of reflection in its own right. Frank, for instance, discusses the significance of *just listening* to others as part of the communal formation of meaning (2001). Such listening has intercorporeal and intersubjective dimensions that together form the bridges that one embodied self traverses to the other.

In tai chi, an example of the intercorporeal aspect this dialogue, or *listening,* is the practice of *adhering and following* the bodily movements and energy of the other, so that one can yield or counter the other, depending on the circumstances (Jwing-Ming, 1999, 15–23). But, according to tai chi masters, adhering and following only occur when one develops *skin feeling* and *listening energy* (18). This intercorporeal tuning into the other finds a parallel in Merleau-Ponty's notion of the intercorporeality that is an essential component of reflectively constructed intersubjectivity. Merleau-Ponty notes "as the parts of my body together comprise a system, so my body and the other's are one whole, two sides of one and the same phenomenon" (1945/1962, 354). Here, the "body proper is a *premonition* of the other" (1964, 175, emphasis added). It is the sense of the other that one tunes into in the *listening* that is part of any dialogue, verbal or nonverbal. Schutz, in "Making Music Together" (1964a) and "Mozart and the Philosophers" (1964b), also notes that the "sharing of the other's flux of experience in inner time, this living through a vivid presence in common . . . constitutes the mutual tuning-in relationship, the 'We'" (1964a, 173). Through flexible rootedness and balance in the ways in which we inhabit the world we already embody, we are enabled to make well-being possible. In interacting with others, whether as sociological researchers or simply as everyday people, we are capable of complex and nuanced understandings of who we are. Entering and interpreting others' worlds, or standing in their shoes, as a modality of reflective sociological practice, can be profoundly enhanced by listening to our own and others' breath.

NOTES

1. *Bracketing* refers to an intentional effort to suspend temporarily one's knowledge, judgments, and beliefs about the meaning that accompanies the lived experience of a particular person, place, event, or thing. The purpose is to hold in abeyance

what one knows in order to observe its construction in and by one's mental and embodied experience. One might say that the purpose is to witness the birth of the meaning of an experience that one would just ordinarily take for granted.

2. In adapting Merleau-Ponty's notions of the habitual body and intercorporeality to sociology, Ostrow (1990) recommended *social sensitivity*. This denotes the way in which the typical becomes habitually embodied so as to prethematically orient one to one's world. This sensitivity builds on Merleau-Ponty's notion that *I am my body* and that *the body is the medium by which I know and express my relation to the world*. Social sensitivity is a distinct advance over Schutz's notion of the *dual mediacy* as the means by which I know the other; dual mediacy is a combination of typifications of the other's interior life with an "immediate experience of his exterior" (Schutz and Luckmann, 1989, 114). Here, knowing the other relies primarily on reflection on the other via typified categories. This passes over the intercorporeal, lived sense that one has of the other preceding categorization.

3. For a related essay, see Donald N. Levine's (1990) "Martial Arts as a Resource for Liberal Education: The Case of Aikido." The difference between this essay and Levine's is the extent to which this essay engages specific themes in phenomenological sociology.

REFERENCES

Berger, Peter L., and Thomas Luckmann. (1966/1967) *The Social Construction of Reality: A Treatise in the Sociology of Knowledge*. New York: Anchor Books.

Bloch, Charlotte. (2000) Flow: Beyond Fluidity and Rigidity. A Phenomenological Investigation. *Human Studies, 23*, 43–61.

Frank, Arthur. (2001) Experiencing Illness Through Storytelling. In S. K. Toombs (Ed.), *Handbook of Phenomenology and Medicine* (229–45). Dordrecht, The Netherlands: Kluwer Academic.

Garfinkel, Harold. (1967) *Studies in Ethnomethodology*. Englewood Cliffs, NJ: Prentice Hall.

Jwing-Ming, Yang. (1999) *Tai Chi Secrets of the Ancient Masters*. Boston: YMAA Publication Center.

LaFountain, Marc J. (1992) Social Sensitivity [review of the book *Social Sensitivity*]. *Phenomenology and the Human Sciences, 17*, 10–17.

Leder, Drew. (1990) *The Absent Body*. Chicago: University of Chicago Press.

Lengermann, Patricia M., and Jill Niebrugge. (1995) Intersubjectivity and Domination: A Feminist Investigation of the Sociology of Alfred Schutz. *Human Studies, 13*, 25–36.

Levine, Donald N. (1990) Martial Arts as a Resource for Liberal Education: The Case of Aikido. In M. Featherstone, M. Hepworth, and B. S. Turner (Eds.), *The Body: Social Process and Cultural Theory* (209–24). Thousand Oaks, CA: Sage.

Lowenthal, Wolfe. (1993) *There Are No Secrets—Professor Cheng Man-ch'ing and His Tai Chi Chuan*. Berkeley, CA: North Atlantic Books.

McGrane, Bernard. (1994) *The Un-TV and the 10 MPH Car: Experiments in Personal Freedom and Everyday Life*. Fort Bragg, CA: The Small Press.

Merleau-Ponty, Maurice. (1945/1962) *Phenomenology of Perception.* (C. Smith, Trans.) London: Routledge & Kegan Paul.

———. (1964) *Signs* (R. McCleary, Trans.) Evanston, IL: Northwestern University Press.

Ostrow, James. (1990) *Social Sensitivity: A Study of Habit and Experience.* Albany: State University of New York Press.

Rehorick, David. (1986) Shaking the Foundations of the Lifeworld: A Phenomenological Account of an Earthquake Experience. *Human Studies, 9,* 379–91.

Schutz, Alfred. (1964a) Making Music Together: A Study in Social Relationship. In A. Schutz, *Collected Papers, vol. II: Studies in Social Theory* (159–78; A. Broderson, Ed.). The Hague, The Netherlands: Martinus Nijhoff.

———. (1964b) Mozart and the Philosophers. In A. Schutz, *Collected Papers, vol. II: Studies in Social Theory* (179–200; A. Broderson, Ed.). The Hague, The Netherlands: Martinus Nijhoff.

———. (1964c) The Stranger: An Essay in Social Psychology. In A. Schutz, *Collected Papers, vol. II: Studies in Social Theory* (91–105; A. Broderson, Ed.). The Hague, The Netherlands: Martinus Nijhoff.

———. (1971) On Multiple Realities. In A. Schutz, *Collected Papers, vol. I: The Problem of Social Reality* (207–59; H. van Breda, Ed.). The Hague, The Netherlands: Martinus Nijhoff.

Schutz, Alfred, and Thomas Luckmann. (1989) The Boundaries of Experience and the Boundary Crossings: Communication in the Life-World. In A. Schutz and T. Luckmann (Eds.), *The Structures of the Life-World, vol. II* (99–157). Evanston, IL: Northwestern University Press.

Seamon, David. (1979) *The Geography of the Lifeworld: Movement, Rest and Encounter.* London: Croom Helm.

Toombs, S. Kay. (2001) Reflections on Bodily Change: The Lived Experience of Disability. In S. K. Toombs (Ed.), *Handbook of Phenomenology and Medicine* (247–61). Dordrecht, The Netherlands: Kluwer Academic.

Young, Iris M. (1990) Throwing Like a Girl: A Phenomenology of Feminine Body Comportment, Motility, and Spatiality. In I. M. Young (Ed.), *Throwing Like a Girl and Other Essays in Feminist Philosophy and Social Theory* (141–59). Bloomington: Indiana University Press.

.

12

Intentionality in Action

Teaching Artists Phenomenology

David B. Haddad

For years, a subtle, persistent set of questions troubled me. Is it possible for me, as a mature, creative adult, to learn a truly new way of seeing things? Is there a reliable decision-making method that I can master? Can I take into account a given state of affairs, deliberately approach it with my whole being, and spontaneously discover the best course of action?

At the time that I felt these questions most keenly, I was a principal in the securities industry with fourteen years under my belt. I was assigned, in turn, to underwriting, trading, and compliance. It was a fast-paced world where many important decisions were made daily. While building my career, I often participated in management's critical decision-making. Sometimes, to my chagrin, the wrong strategy would be voted in. Unfortunately, I found myself at a loss to make safer, surer courses of action compelling enough to be adopted by my fellow company officers. This frustrated me, and I was ultimately motivated to look again to discover new ways of seeing, processing, and coming to decisions. My drive came not from the desire for financial success; rather, it was to avoid the costly, recurring, self-destructive errors in judgment that I observed within high-stakes, complex business settings.

If I could find the right methods, I reasoned, I could pass them on to others. But adequate tools to test the idea seemed to elude me as long as I limited my search to information sources in the financial industry. I felt that, unless I was serious enough about the question to return to school, I would never have a satisfactory answer. So I did. I was determined to find whatever the best of the best had to say in the matter. Scholars in organizational psychology devoted their lives to addressing the questions of decision-making and change; surely, they had some success. I wanted to know their solutions, no matter how deep; I would take their theories and apply what they prescribed in everyday language to the real-world problems that I experienced. Thus, I decided, at midlife, to pursue a Ph.D. My target was not just knowledge but, if possible, an application of the learning to my own daily concerns.

I carefully reviewed the leading schools, and finally settled on Fielding Graduate University. There, I would have the flexibility I needed, as a midlife professional, to search out my questions under the best academic guidance, but without disrupting my entire life by pulling up stakes, concluding commitments to my community, and moving my family to a residential school. I found Fielding to be a perfect fit for my independent, self-directed approach to work.

The midlife financial professional-turned-doctoral student now sought to satisfy the abiding question: Can I access and apply renewable insight in a regular, reliable manner? My endeavor was on behalf of the young man in me, who strived for, but never found, a dependable, resilient method of decision-making. This effort was also for the youth still alive in me, a remnant of innocence that believed deep knowledge could not harm.

If I needed to get a grip on valuable insights that could smooth the troubled paths of business relationships, I reasoned, perhaps others, too, may value learning them. I had already read a breadth of self-help and how-to books, but each seemed to add just another layer of understanding over my own. Superimposing one more layer of someone else's meanings to my life didn't seem to solve anything. The intermediate quality of their systems of self-improvement only burdened me with a new set of dynamics to track.

After nearly a year of reviewing more scholarly literature on human consciousness, I found myself reading a great deal of phenomenology, which delves beneath the complex concepts of psychology. Known to philosophers and scholars for the past one hundred years, phenomenology is more than philosophy; it is a *method of knowing* based in tangible human experience. What drew me further into phenomenology was its fundamental aim: questioning the structure and dynamics of intentionality, the very heart of human consciousness. Once on this path, I discovered a means for logical, comprehensive investigation that applies to the real world of experience. Phenomenology is a global approach to the abundantly detailed meaning-making capacity generated in human relationships.

The literature offers a rich orientation toward the nature of being and time, knowledge and perception, and, most of all, relationships. Phenomenology entails scrupulously defined thinking. Its methods are simultaneously razor sharp, yet generously allow for the unavoidable ambiguities of life. I needed this. Its thoroughness instilled confidence. I familiarized myself with the methods of phenomenology, which promised to reach down to the concrete level where I really lived, unlike anything I had tried before.

Thinking in phenomenological terms immediately raised another obstacle. Assuming that I could access the information, the real work boiled down to translating scholarly methods into everyday language so that I could apply them in practice. The literature of phenomenology had been written by and for scholars, philosophers, and phenomenologists, not artists, business professionals, or tradespeople. Nevertheless, I felt fairly certain that these dense instructions could be made more accessible to the vast majority of people unschooled in them.

To test whether I could connect abstract phenomenological language and concepts with actual, everyday dialogue, I designed a research method to engage participants who had no background in phenomenology. I felt that I could get past the challenging language and assist them in learning how to write phenomenological protocols, which are rich descriptions of immediate experience. I could, then, determine whether writing such protocols was beneficial to them, especially if it helped them with their work.

THE STUDY: AN EXPERIMENT IN APPLIED PHENOMENOLOGY

I invited twelve artists to collaborate with me as research participants. They ranged in age from mid-thirties to late sixties. Most were white, middle-class Americans with a variety of ethnic and religious backgrounds. None had been educated beyond the masters' level and none was schooled in phenomenology. All were artists or performers.

I assumed certain things about an artist's motivation. Artists, more than others, experience a dissatisfaction with life that they confront, through art, rather than evade or ignore. Their responses to life's issues seem to come out of an exigency, an urgent need to respond. In their acts of responding to a given state of affairs, they somehow manage to relieve the pressures of their perceptions of life through creative expression. I interpreted the creative quality of that response to mean that they had mustered a second important attribute: the courage to attempt unique solutions to life's challenges. Furthermore, I believed that their attempts were undertaken with some degree of faith that their efforts would somehow pay off. That blended motivation, regardless of the relative success of prior efforts, was evidence of the tenacity required to finish the process of writing phenomenological protocols about their art. This was the task I presented to them. Here, one participant's process illustrates the method. An actual application is important; to view through another's experience helps to describe phenomenology in action.

The first four of five data-gathering sessions required textual responses. For the fifth session, the final synthesis, I offered an optional medium of communication; the participants were free to choose text or make use of their own artistic craftsmanship. Half of them opted for the artistic alternative. From twelve participants, I received final syntheses in the forms of a painting, a collage, and four sculptures. Their artistic objects were then interpreted to fill in any gaps remaining after the psychological phase. From the dozen participants came a wide range of output. Here, one illustration (due to space limitations) highlights the difficulty of communicating the method, but that it is accessible and of value for artists.

My question revolved around two concepts coupled with a task: the nature of perception, the real world perceived, and the accessibility of the phenomenological method outlined by Edmund Husserl in *Ideas I* (1913/ 1982, §§31–33). Further iterations of phenomenological protocols, such as Clark Moustakas's (1994) and Max van Manen's (1990), have added clarity and texture to Husserl's method. My goal was to instruct artists with no prior knowledge of phenomenology to write and think about their work using the techniques of writing protocols, and work with them using bracketing, imaginative variations, and other phenomenological techniques.

The steps in my application of the phenomenological reduction are as follows:

1. Initiate an act of intentionality simply by making a spontaneous choice. Participants were urged to make their choice about a *future* state of affairs.
2. Describe your choice in the fullest possible detail. To assist the participants, I encouraged them to base their descriptions on a range of existential categories. I asked them to describe their intentional act in terms of time, space, the body, and their relationships to others. Meditation develops most of its content by applying these existential prompts.
3. Next was the clustering phase, to cluster meanings, to identify and isolate themes. Phrases, sentences, even whole paragraphs, of rich description were brought together into concentrations of like thoughts. Then we mined their horizontal qualities. Each horizon of the meditation was an aspect of the meaning within the overall meditation. Each was considered on its own merits, in isolation from the rest, so that its full significance could be felt and explored. Once exploration of horizons begins, one quickly discovers their open-endedness. Horizons of meaning possess inexhaustible qualities.
4. Next, we inverted the contents of the meditation. By subjecting the results gained to playfully upturned, imaginative reversals and polarities, we were able to shake ourselves out of any residual linear think-

ing and consider the radical breadth still buried in the original act of intentionality.

5. Finally, we reassessed and condensed the entire meditation into a final synthesis. Whereas all of the above steps were carried out in writing, only the final synthesis was open to artistic rather than textual rendering.

Together, we bracketed out everyday taken-for-granted meanings and connotations, which prepared us for a final synthesis. The structural significance of the process was twofold in nature. First was perceiving the naked object of one's consciousness, an intentional act unembellished by the multitude of related, extraneous, distracting preconceptions typically found in one's stock of knowledge. Secondly, bracketing allowed us to clearly behold the authentic nature of the actual external object, person, or state of affairs for what it was. Each session was held in the same location. Some participants invited me into their homes, some their studios, and others their offices. Each situation was private, uninterrupted, and comfortable enough to allow us to focus on the work at hand.

I described the project as a study that I was conducting for my doctoral dissertation, in which their voluntary participation would be appreciated. The only setup I provided for the work that they would do was that it involved five steps. I made it clear that I needed them to respond to my instructions in writing, that our conversations would be recorded, and that strict confidentiality would apply. Each of the participants signed and kept a copy of a release.

I purposely gave the participants very little in preparatory remarks. The study's design presupposed nothing about the participants' capacity to engage with the material. For that reason, the actual engagement of the protocol took place spontaneously, one session at a time. As I delivered the instructions for each successive step, I also handed them a written version to which they could refer thereafter. Collaboration in the creation of a shared understanding began only as each participant indicated that he had grasped the material.

MÖBIUS: AN ILLUSTRATIVE ACCOUNT

Möbius, a pseudonym inspired by his end product, is an Asian-American business consultant, married, in his forties, living in Southern California. Monitoring his progress through the five-session process highlights the dynamics of engaging phenomenology, action research, and hermeneutics. Sometimes, I first emphasized the phenomenological reduction; other times, I centered on our interaction, as we used the action research cycle to shape and reshape the language of my instructions.

Session 1

Möbius was the first participant to plunge into session 1 instructions and spontaneously envision a future state of affairs. Without hesitating, Möbius made his choice and projected his desired state of affairs, casting it in the future perfect tense:

> I *will have learned* how to pace myself throughout the day and schedule my tasks so that they get done in such a way that I am proud of what I have done. I *will have felt* pride because I was able to discipline myself to do the things I feel are important for my well-being and happiness. (emphasis added)

Möbius's choice constituted an intentional act, one that he could explore in search of its essential features.

Session 2

Building upon this intentional act, we came to pivotal elements beginning in session 2, the phase of rich description. I asked Möbius to write, as fully detailed as he could. Offering a bit of structure around which to form richly detailed description, I introduced Möbius to the following existential prompts: space and environment, time and temporality, the experience of his lived body, and what happened when he encountered "the Other." He based his writings on a blend of the choices he had made with these four prompts. The session soon became complicated; he balked, critically challenging the language I used to highlight the existential prompts. On second look, it was not difficult for me to see why. The meaning behind the text of the meditation was abstract and unclear. I began with a rather dry and awkward explanation of how to proceed:

> Richly describe it [the intentional projection] in as great detail as possible using the four existentials. As a guide to reflection, use these four prompts: (a) the quality of your lived space, viewing both *forest* and *trees*; (b) your body as a lived object; (c) temporality and the velocity of time; (d) the lived other, resulting in transcendent conversational relations that lift you out of yourself, so to speak. You rediscover meanings, purpose, and grounds for living in the company of others.

As spoken instructions, it sounded like a cold command, not a warm invitation. Considered in print, the conceptual quality of the language lent precision, compactness, and a certain forcefulness. Had Möbius had prior exposure to the method of phenomenological reduction, or come to the task with more of an aptitude for abstractions, there may have been less of a problem. But for him, the protocol instructions lacked concrete qualities, leaving him disengaged. The last thing I wanted was to find that language had become a barrier to learning. To re-engage, we needed to develop new wording.

We made minor modifications in wording each of the four existentials. On the issue of temporality and the velocity of time, however, our collaboration was especially challenging. In order to stimulate a sense of the breadth of temporality, I suggested the possibility of some distinct manner in which people are *gaited* to their generation, a sort of collegial locking of elbows with the spirit of the times.

The breadth of these new instructions opened a path of accessibility. When I used the terms *rhythm, tempo, pace,* and *gait,* Möbius began to perceive, with greater ease and transparency, the personal implications of inner-time consciousness. Möbius navigated a seesaw tension between pleasure and self-discipline, and reassessed his time management skills:

> I will have organized my workspace so it supports whatever I am doing. . . . I will have set a schedule for routine things. . . . I will have realized that surfing the web can be horribly time consuming. I will have finished the final editing of my series of special reports. . . . I will have planned what I will do the next day and have it typed in a Word file. . . . I will have known at all times what my priorities were and will have worked on the most important things. I will have learned from this planning [that] being absolutely rigid with my schedule is not the best way to go. I will have learned that being flexible is a great skill to possess. . . . I will have felt a tremendous sense of accomplishment by doing this.

As hoped, our revised protocol language lent new texture to his writing. What, at first, seemed obscure soon changed, reinvigorating his grasp of the protocol. Language that began as merely skeletal and formulaic gained fuller anatomy and a more resilient structure, eventually leading to an exercise that was vibrant and accessible.

Session 3

Session 3 involved *horizons* and *clustering*. I worked with Möbius through the description of horizons and a process of clustering multiple components of the experience. Möbius produced themes of productivity, ritual, organization, prioritization, awareness, and goal setting:

> I'm seeing that the underlying theme to all of this is self-discipline. I tend to get distracted and do the things I like to do or are pleasurable. . . . Is there some way to develop this discipline? Is there some way I can make the task more pleasurable? Will thinking about how good I will feel at the completion of the task give me the proper motivation?

Session 4

Continuing his meditation with session 4, I presented Möbius with the exercise of imaginative variation. This was a special treatment of the themed clusters he had collected in session 3. I asked Möbius to reexamine the themes on which he had worked so hard to excavate. The task was to vary the frames of reference in which he contained the themes, on a scale from mild to radical variation, even to the point of completely inverting the contents of the meditation.

The goal of subjecting the meditation's results to playfully upturned, imaginative reversals and polarities is to shake oneself out of linear thinking, to consider afresh the more radical breadth hidden within the original intentional act. Yet this is easier said than done. Möbius's challenge to my instructions forced me to find another way to express the meaning and intent of Edmund Husserl's writings.

The very concept that I proposed in session 4 seemed alien to Möbius's way of thinking. I asked him to consider his self-identified issues of awareness, self-discipline, and pleasure from entirely new vantage points. I prepared him for the work of the session by drawing upon a suggestion from Moustakas (1994): to employ polarities and reversals, and approach the phenomenon from divergent perspectives. In short, he was asked to set aside the familiar and think anew.

This abstract language fell on deaf ears. We reworked the instructions again. After some effort, we finally substituted new phrasing: "Use all of your intellectual and emotional capacities, your imagination, and intuition." This replaced the jargon of the original language—"Adjust and catalyze the frames of reference"—which required comprehension of technical constructions such as *catalyze* and *frames of reference*, whereas the new instruction used common words. The revised language also seemed to communicate better the challenging personal effort required in session 4. Further editing replaced phrases such as "mundane existence is no longer central" and "anything whatever becomes possible" with this directive: "Free your mind and intuition. Use the furthest limits of your imagination. Look for taboos, or at least welcome them as signals if they arise."

One of our goals, along with accessing the phenomenological reduction, was collaboration to find active, stimulating language that remained true to the intent of each session. Accepting Möbius's objections, I sought out wording that brought the clarity cited above, where the source material was deemed too conceptual, jargonistic, or vague. A livelier, more familiar set of expressions radiated a natural, more human feel in place of what otherwise sounded obscurely scientific and thus dead or intimidating. A sample of Möbius's writing illustrates how he worked through session 4:

> I have self-discipline for the things I love to do. For example, when I'm writing a speech I'll just do it and it becomes enjoyable. Self-discipline and pleasure, hmmm, seems like a contradiction in terms. What I'm seeing in myself is the ability to put a lot of concentration and energy into things I enjoy. If the enjoyment isn't there, it's difficult for me to put the concentration and energy into it.

Three pages later, Möbius was still working through session 4, but his evaluation of his intentional act about pleasure and self-discipline had evolved:

> Going off on another path here. Who has been really into pleasure and yet self-discipline? Oooh, just had an interesting thought. Is self-discipline in itself pleasurable? Maybe a better question would be how to make self-discipline pleasurable.

His intermediate meditations and final summary provide a foretaste of Möbius's final synthesis:

> This assignment seems to be the most difficult of all. What did Dave say about the taboos? Look for them or at least welcome them when they show up. Pain and pleasure. Ooops! Was that a Freudian slip? I meant to say self-discipline and pleasure. Maybe that's why my mind is rejecting a lot of these ideas. Pain and pleasure. Organisms spend their lives moving towards pleasure and moving away from pain. If I'm associating pain with self-discipline I get caught in a contradiction. . . .
>
> *Summary*: I've linked self-discipline with pleasure. I use (a) awareness, (b) curiosity about whether it is possible to lower self-discipline to do a certain task, (c) stream-of-consciousness, and (d) anticipation of discovery to transform non-pleasurable self-discipline into pleasurable self-discipline.

Möbius's imaginative variations reveal a breakthrough in understanding. No longer was he embedded in his internal conflict about self-discipline. He perceived the object of his consciousness, the state of affairs at which his intentional act was aimed. Through the process, he learned how to unhitch his subconscious, negative association with self-discipline, and consciously rehitch it to a powerfully positive one: pleasure. It took several weeks and awareness of what he was doing—awareness discovered through his textual exercises—until Möbius was freed from his self-defeating habit of mind.

Our teamwork in recasting the language brought Möbius relief. He experienced a personal advance in his inner life. Simultaneously, his insight affected his day-to-day professional behavior.

Session 5

Möbius's final synthesis is the paper sculpture pictured here (Haddad, 2002, 148):

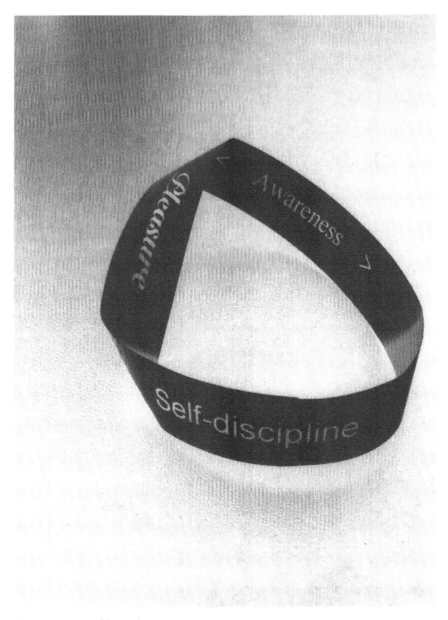

Figure 12.1. Möbius Strip

Expressing his final synthesis in a paper sculpture, rather than text alone, he presented me with a Möbius strip. Representing flow and deep movement, the strip indicated that he had resolved the internal conflict with which he had struggled from the beginning. The strip depicted a perpetual meaning continuum, flowing in both directions out of *awareness*. Following the arrows indicating the movement of his awareness, the first theme of his meditation was made explicit: *self-discipline*. Moving in the opposite direction, the second recurring theme was made explicit: *pleasure*. The last part of our work together involved interpreting his final synthesis.

Interpretation

A Möbius strip is a physical reality that defies logic. It is a flat surface possessing only one edge and only one side. Rendering his deep, conflicted, yet positive motivations with this ingenious device, Möbius simultaneously separated and united the distinct meanings that flowed through him. He was able to perceive, and ultimately reconcile, what previously had seemed to him to be abiding, irreconcilable drives. He did so in an artistic, unconventional, but perfectly acceptable manner. The twist of the Möbius strip depicted the reconciliation clearly and concretely.

He had accessed the protocol. We had successfully collaborated to make it possible. His final work shows both aspects of the lifeworld. On one hand, he had a powerful conceptual breakthrough. His initial intentional act, worked through the steps of our meditation, resolved an important motivational roadblock. On the other hand, he was newly empowered to engage fully with his real, external world, the world that presented him with what he first perceived as a conundrum that required self-discipline when he wanted, instead, to revel in pleasure.

Möbius compounded the effect of our study by using his own powers of mind as applied to his intentional object. His intentional act began with a focus on the mundane procedures of his work environment. The protocol, however, quickly opened new horizons to the functional dynamics of his mind and its predisposed relationship to his surrounding world. Möbius was able to see how he had come to crossed purposes within himself. Once the dynamics of his internal dialogue became evident, he was empowered to unravel the motivational knot that had short-circuited a portion of his joy.

PERSONAL INSIGHTS AND REFLECTIVE UNDERSTANDINGS

My first discovery confirmed what I had hoped: that individuals without any background whatsoever in phenomenology can engage it meaningfully.

I found that nine of the twelve participants were able to learn how to do the phenomenological reduction. They were able to apply the method from start to finish without first having to digest a vast new vocabulary. The depth of their participation was evidenced by the results. Each manifested a beginner's eager grasp of the material.

I, too, experienced a breakthrough in constructing new language that made the phenomenological reduction an accessible method for a business professional. As a researcher and collaborator, I was able to synthesize a more appropriate instrument, one formed with everyday language. What would have otherwise escaped me, I felt, now could be passed on more easily to other participants.

A second discovery involved the tension between modifying the protocol language and remaining faithful to the method's original intent. When my instructions were not immediately clear, I encouraged the participants to help me. With their help, I continued to tailor new language to suit their temperaments and outlooks. We collaborated on several innovative substitutions to the protocol language. As we made substitutions, I continued to look at the original texts to ensure that the revised wording remained consonant. Keeping the use of language flexible and open for modification enabled us to revise and, in the participants' minds, greatly improve access to the method. The end product was a refined, rigorously edited guide, a *phenomenological method in modern English*, if you will, faithful to the spirit and intent of the original translated writings of Edmund Husserl.

A final discovery was a new appreciation, on my part, of what phenomenology calls the *lifeworld*. I recognized that my natural research orientation favors the world of ideas over the world of concrete reality. But the work of investigating my participants' textual and artistic renderings of consciousness gradually expanded my view. I was compelled to examine, interpret, and reexamine the products of their meditations. As a result, I was able to strike a healthier balance between my preference for theoretical abstractions and the concrete lifeworld.

Briefly, the principle of the lifeworld is two things, simultaneously. It is the creative powers of the subject, the individual, at work in the world from her unique perspective. It is a cycle of simple and complex acts of intentionality, out of which meaning-making between the person and his surrounding social and material environment builds up over time. But it is much more than a string of acts of intentionality. The lifeworld is the real, concrete surrounding world of objects, states of affairs, and other people. The lifeworld irrevocably entwines one's powers of mind—that is, intentionality and meaning-making—with external, enduring social existence. In short, the lifeworld is the world with which the individual has to deal. It is intersubjectively verifiable and, thus, a place where minds meet.

Intersubjectivity is the bridge that makes human contact possible at its deepest levels. The concrete external world was reconstituted, for me, as the necessary correlate of thought. After all, what is thought without action? Taken together, these discoveries strongly suggest that a deep and powerful method of knowledge is within reach of virtually anyone. Why is that important? Because the ways in which individuals go about knowing their worlds, the philosophies they bring to experience, determine in large part what meanings can be taken away.

The advantage of using phenomenology is, first, a deepening of one's inner emotional and intellectual grasp of life's details. Second, the phenomenological protocol significantly clarifies and qualifies the dynamics that undergird personal interaction in the external world, one's lifeworld. This dual action helps prevent experience and thought from outpacing one another. The reduction provides a method by which a practitioner can experience the syncopated relationship of thought and action as meaningful, synchronous harmony.

The relationship between thought and action may be seen as a gap. Traversing that gap links my solitary life to the concrete social world around me. In this case, the gap is the distance over which life and meaning—in the form of intentionality—flow from me to my physical-social surround and back again. As life and meaning flow day by day, my lifeworld takes shape. How deep are the meanings made? As deep as I wish to plumb. The beauty is that deeper meaning and more durable empowerment await me as both a solitary individual and one member among many in the community.

After several years of coaching and consulting, I returned to the financial industry. I continue to coach colleagues and clients who elect it, by introducing them to the phenomenological protocol. The phenomenological protocol has proven to be a reliable, systematic approach that reinvigorates one's insight, affords new breakthroughs, and endows the client with enduring empowerment to achieve one's desired goals. The phenomenological reduction would be the *magic bullet* for which business professionals hunt, were it not such a demanding process. The client's hard work, however, pays off. It is not unusual for a client to discover that his priorities get rearranged.

My clients have changed their lives for the better through this reinvigorated, phenomenologically inspired, collaborative coaching process. For example, a single mother and successful real estate professional has moved from Portland, Oregon, to Krakow, Poland, for a year. Her goals, which came to light after a few sessions of phenomenological exercises, called for direct involvement housing orphaned children, teaching illiterate women to read, and writing a book. Another client was on the verge of acquiring control of a $50 million automotive supplier and merging it with a $300 million manufacturer, while simultaneously salvaging his marriage of fifteen years. Both clients are beneficiaries of the phenomenological protocol.

As a protocol coach, I get clients to look past the immediate appearances of their circumstances to explore the underlying dynamics of their life-world. I hold up a mirror, as it were, to let them see their relationships anew, and the dynamics that ground them in those relationships, holding them accountable for their own perceptions in a disciplined spirit of good faith. For those who decline coaching, I suggest several accessible books that offer, step by step, the process described here.

Human consciousness is not meant to be dominated by circumstances. My study of phenomenology and application of the phenomenological protocols offer promise and hope.

REFERENCES

Droysen, Johann G. (1967) *Outline of the Principles of History.* New York: Howard Fertig.

Haddad, David B. (2002) *Intentionality as an Instrument in Action Research.* Unpublished Ph.D. Dissertation. Santa Barbara, CA: Fielding Graduate Institute.

Husserl, Edmund. (1982) *Ideas Pertaining to a Pure Phenomenology and to a Phenomenological Philosophy: First Book* (F. Kersten, Trans.). The Hague, The Netherlands: Martinus Nijhoff.

Kegan, Robert. (1994) *In Over Our Heads: The Mental Demands of Modern Life.* Cambridge, MA: Harvard University Press.

Lewin, Kurt. (1946) Action Research and Minority Problems. *Journal of Social Issues,* 2(4), 34–36.

Lewis, C. S. (1947) *Miracles: A Preliminary Study.* New York: Macmillan.

Moustakas, Clark E. (1994) *Phenomenological Research Methods.* Thousand Oaks, CA: Sage.

Schutz, Alfred. (1970) *On Phenomenology and Social Relations.* Chicago: University of Chicago Press.

van Manen, Max. (1990) *Researching Lived Experience.* London, Ontario, Canada: Althouse Press.

Zahavi, Dan. (2003) *Husserl's Phenomenology: Cultural Memory in the Present.* Palo Alto, CA: Stanford University Press.

13

Chasing Transcendence

Experiencing Magic Moments in Jazz Improvisation

Steven C. Jeddeloh

This chapter describes my exploration of the experience I call the *magic moment*: the transcendent or peak moment as experienced by jazz musicians. The following narrative offers a glimpse into my own lifeworld as a jazz musician experiencing a magic moment in a jazz performance.

> I was sitting in with a group of jazz musicians assembled in orderly rows, greatly anticipating the leap from a classical context to a jazz improvisation. The odds of getting to where we wished to go were against us. We assembled as a music class, not as a group of experienced improvisers. The leader was a classically trained trumpet player. He obviously knew his way around a musical score and definitely had the will, desire, and excitement for delving into a jazz experience—but he had no experience playing jazz, let alone leading a jazz group.
>
> Out of twenty musicians, perhaps three had improvisation experience. I certainly wasn't one of the three, but I was there with desire, curiosity, passion and lots of trepidation. We read the chart, made music and began the journey to learn and experience the art of playing jazz, of improvisation and, hopefully, of making a little magic. As part of that first session we were each to take a solo, a stab at improvisation in a simple, predictable system of chord modulations.
>
> As my solo approached, I vacillated between sheer terror and a sort of blissful connection to the musical flow. When I began my solo, I had a sense of letting go of the chart and the way the music was written, and I surrendered to the flow of the music. In a way, I lost consciousness except consciousness of the rhythm and tones of the musical world in which I was floating. I lost track of the written music, the instrument, my "self," time, and my surroundings.
>
> I soloed long past my prescribed section and played until my sense of what I was playing seemed naturally to finish its course. I woke up. The rest of the

musicians had already stopped playing. My terror returned. My first sense was that I had just committed a heinous crime, a musical murder in the first degree. On the contrary, the expressions I first took as anger or disgust were looks of awe and wonder. There were cheers such that one would hear upon scoring the winning point in a championship game. (Jeddeloh, 2001, 177)

This experience occurred almost thirty years ago, yet, in my mind, the event is still as vivid as if it happened yesterday. I have always been fascinated and mystified by what occurred in that session, and have never been able to explain it, nor did I necessarily want to do so, for fear of it losing some of its magic. Since that performance, I have heard others' descriptions of experiences that seem to have similar, life-changing impact, experiences encountered in a wide variety of environments and disciplines: work, spirituality, and play, as an individual, and while in relationship with others.

Transcendent experiences are highly revered, mysterious, and magical facets of the human experience. Most of us experience *magic moments* during intense experiences such as exercise, childbirth, spiritual acts, love, music-making, artistic creation, and work. A transcendent experience can be described as an event in time experienced by an individual and/or a group, a conscious knowing of something "boundless and limitless," beyond one's conscious grasp and which "surpasses human capacities" (Roy, 2001, xi). It is thought of as outside of day-to-day life and a "powerful emersion into a transformed unity" (Greeley, 1974, 24). There is a sense of connecting with something that lies beyond everyday control, power, or understanding.

Transcendent-state intensity ranges from states of seeming deep sleep to wide-awake, conscious awareness, from the dreamlike to the lucid, from relaxation to intense arousal, from total nothingness to inspired creativity, from reality to hallucination, and/or from angst to ecstasy. Most descriptions note these experiences as momentary and fleeting, yet the post-transcendent aftereffect is often said to linger as a feeling of positive emotion and/or enlightenment (Laski, 1961, 6). The subjective nature of the experience makes the lasting effects quite individualistic. According to Laski, some of the common characteristics include a profound loss of self, while experiencing a sense of unity or interconnectedness, clarity of perception, and a loss of the sense of external time, space, worldliness, and individual limitations (444–69). At the same time, there is a sense of increased joy, love, ecstasy, release, as well as augmented physical and mental capabilities. The preparatory phase may be characterized by such feelings as intense inner conflict, despair, and discomfort. The transcendence period is characterized by an altered state of consciousness that includes a feeling of oneness, illumination, vision, and ecstasy. This is followed by a period of shifting, characterized by the questions *What just happened?* and *What does it mean?*

Jazz musicians describe feelings of being completely focused and inspired, similar to the experience of a scientist having a *eureka* experience, performing far beyond their normal capacity. The musicians' sense of time often slows so that it feels as if the music and the play are not as fast or furious as they really are, allowing more of what they have inside to come out. Because the improvising musician is composing in play, the entire musical concept, with all the harmonic changes, is grasped at once, making the improvisation seem similar to flowing waves and textures rather than a series of notes. Musicians talk about inspirational jazz performers who have gone before, whose riffs they have practiced and copied, embedding them in memory.

To explore the phenomenon of magic moments, I was drawn to the literature documenting what is known about the inner workings of body-mind and consciousness. I explored music theory and psychology to understand the role that music plays in this magic-moment experience. I explored how the relationship between the self and other impacts this experience. And I explored phenomenological method relating to transcendent experience. Below, I highlight only my research into the phenomenological stream of published research.

JAZZ IMPROVISATION AS PHENOMENOLOGICAL METHOD

The nature of musical time is defined by duration—not so much the pulse or notes as the spaces between. Rhythm engages and invites us in to entrain, not reacting to the rhythm as we do with most stimuli, but coupling with it as a synchronized, communal rhythm. The synchronized, mutual presence of *durée*, Henri Bergson's notion, is a space where the explicit nature of music fades away, where participants lose their sense of self and couple with others in their own, yet mutual, inner time (1913/2001, 1998). The root of this implicitness is time defined by the rhythm and meter of the music and the internal body-mind rhythms of the participants.

The act of jazz improvisation is a phenomenological method of reflecting within what Alfred Schutz calls the *we-relationship*, reducing the melody of a song to its basic melodic form and using creative variation to take that melody and create new meaning (1967, 167). This musical phenomenological method may also be likened to the Buddhist method of *Samatha*, or mindfulness and introspection, sustaining the recollection of an image, observing it while taking the role as a "disinterested spectator," maintaining it without "excitation" or "laxity," but a "serene attentional state" (Wallace, 1999, 97, 176). This maintaining and examining an image is similar to Husserl's *phenomenological reduction*, and his notion of *epoche*, "the gesture of suspension with regard to the habitual course of one's thoughts brought about by an interruption of their continuous flowing" (Depraz, 1999, 99).

The Husserlian idea of *eidetic reduction* is to reduce an object to its lowest form, its concrete experience, and cause us to question our attachment to fact, which, to Husserl, was limited to the actualization of one possibility alone. The basic experience, on the other hand, is rich and full of all kinds of potentialities inherent in subjectivity: in this case, creative variation (Depraz, 1999, 101). Samatha mindfulness, similarly, advocates an introspective examination of the image of an *object*, shifting from focus on the object to the experience of the object, recalling associated subjective experiences. This practice provides a way to examine both the object and the subjective experience. Mindful focusing on the motif or initial melody, examining it and staying focused on it as the object, yet allowing the subjective, the experiential, to arise in the play, and shifting from the object to the subjective recollection of it in the span of about ten milliseconds constructs the improvisation (Wallace, 1999, 177). According to musicians, the more the attachments are *let go*, the better the play. The transcendent state, when achieved in improvised play, finds the mindful musician at once focused (in the Samathic tradition) and introspective (aware of retrospective experience), providing a sort of subject-object field of visual (image) experience. An example is a musician fueled by a past emotional trauma while simultaneously focusing on the musical object (motif) of the song.

THE PERFORMANCE LIFEWORLD

The importance of relationship in the music-making cannot be overemphasized, with critical relationships found between musicians, the musician and the instrument, and the ensemble and the listeners. Developing community between musicians, the composer, and the listeners creates the space for a magic moment to occur. A socially constructed jazz music culture is created within this community, which embodies the cultural realities brought to the community by each of the participants. In my research, jazz ensembles were filmed in a variety of environments, including a musician's living room, a larger studio, and a quintet performance at a well-known jazz club with an audience of about thirty-five people (Jeddeloh, 2003). I will describe the group performing in the jazz club environment in more detail to illustrate structures of the musicians' lifeworld.

The quintet consisted of a drummer, bass, piano, and alto and tenor sax players. The musicians had not played together before, so they were relying on their knowledge of the music and local jazz conventions to develop their collaboration. The stage was set up as a semicircle, approximately thirty feet wide at the front, narrowing to fifteen feet at the back. The bass and drummer set up at the back, while the baby grand piano was positioned at the side, facing the other musicians; the two sax players set up in front. The musicians were microphoned, with a sound person mixing the audio in the back of the room.

The song list was established at the beginning of the evening, all songs with which the players were familiar and arranged so that the music would start out simple and grow in complexity and intensity as the three sets progressed. In the first set, the musicians were *feeling each other out*, testing one another to see how free they were to take risks. By the third set, each was playing flat out, relying on the others to offer support and encouragement.

There were distractions. A loud couple, drinking there before the group assembled, got louder as the music began. Although the musicians described a process of *tuning out* the couple, they talked about them enough afterward to indicate their awareness. As performance intensity increased, the attention of the audience shifted from socializing to engaging with the music. At one intense point, the audience ceased talking altogether, riveted to the group and the soloing alto sax.

COLLECTING DATA: PHENOMENOLOGICAL INSIGHTS THROUGH STIMULATED RECALL

Each ensemble reviewed its videotaped performance, and stopped the tape whenever the musicians wished to describe what they were viewing (for details of research method, see Gass and Mackey, 2000). I audiotaped and transcribed the resulting dialogue. I used the videotapes, the audiotapes, the transcripts, and my notes as the research data.

Bracketing my own theories, I observed the magic moment as if a member of each ensemble. Thus, I became a mystery explorer, partnering with the musicians in a *face-to-face situation*, using dialogue as a method of meaning-making and social construction. I attempted to *get within reach* of direct experience with the musicians, sharing a *community of space and a community of time* where there is *awareness* of each person as a particular individual, where, as Alfred Schutz indicates, "We are growing older together" (1967, 163). My research process was intended to provide a space where the participants and I could explore together.

Jazz improvisation is an example of comingling in the we-relationship, where cominglers are locked in one another's consciousness within a span of time. Jazz musicians must lock into the consciousness of the other musicians to create collaborative meaning. Once the videotaped performance was complete, I invited the participants to join with me, stepping back and reflecting on what happened, withdrawing from the performance relationship to establish a new we-relationship to reflect on the performance, "living in our common stream of consciousness" (Schutz, 1967, 167). I was part of the performance (albeit peripheral) and later accepted as an integral member of the group while sitting in a musician's home, reviewing the videotape, and entering into this group's collaborative consciousness to prod, challenge, and add my own views about what we were seeing.

Musicians used *typifications* to describe their taken-for-granted musical experience. I encouraged them to expand their descriptions further, asking for examples and reactions from the other musicians. These typifications were their commonsense descriptions, using familiar terms to describe or explain the unusual or unexplainable, maintaining the integrity of the natural attitude. Typifications shield us from experience that is beyond our grasp and control, using commonsense language to make the unknown, the unsettling, and unfamiliar more understandable within a world of well-known objects with familiar qualities, keeping our world comfortable and sustainable.

The musicians and I were living in the we-relationship, the common stream of consciousness, with the video providing the *freezing* of the subjective experience for the musicians' reflection upon it (Schutz, 1967, 167). This was an adventure for them, as they had not discussed the magic moment with one another before, other than to indicate the *typical* experience of *hitting a groove* or creating a *flow*. Descriptions inevitably overlapped in meaning, not creating consensus or definitive explanation, but providing similarities and differences to explore. The transcriptions produced hundreds of pages of musician statements, wherein thirteen musicians added their voices and settled into a dialogue, an improvised conversation similar to that witnessed in the actual performances.

Through a process of recording jazz performance, comingling and exploring that performance with musicians, creating meaning through improvised dialogue, and connecting the resulting discoveries with the published research literature, I have given voice and clarity to the magic moment: an intimate, human, lived experience.

DESCRIBING MAGIC MOMENTS: WHAT MUSICIANS SAY

Most of the musicians described their first experience with a magic moment as involving a non-musical, rhythmic, physical activity, such as throwing bales of hay on a farm. The context of the moment was relevant, but not as important as the physical, embodied aspects of the event, enhanced by an extended block of time, a rhythmicity of movement, and a detachment, with concentrated focus on the task and the moment. The magic moment was considered outside of the normal, day-to-day experience: an unexpected, pleasurable, and mysterious event. They described the event using typical language:

Brian (a pseudonym): I remember feeling exhilaration. Where everything was easy and perfect. Throwing bales, getting into a rhythm. It was satisfaction as well as what was happening: accomplishing something worthwhile.

The unknown was drawn into the person's lifeworld and explained by known experience, using typical language.

By experiencing this new, heretofore unknown, event in the person's lifeworld, typifications maintain the individual's sense of maintaining normalcy: "A new experience has been added to the stock-of-experiences-at-hand, but in a way which promotes continuation and contextual closure" (Rehorick, 1986, 384). Similarly, while reviewing one of the videotaped sessions, one musician explained feelings of levitating, weightlessness, and lightness of being, using more scientific language:

Brian: And part of it might be just the wave of vibrations of the sound that travel throughout your whole body, and it gives everything the same kind of vibration.

This typification, and scientific *possibilizing*, is a way to legitimize the unexplainable or rare event: "a way to restore one's balance and 'reground' the self" (385). Having experienced the magic moment earlier on in life, there is a *taken-for-grantedness* of the aspects of the events musicians experienced in music (Schutz and Luckmann, 1973, 6; Zaner, 1981, 168).

Magic-moment sensations are rare, but expected, taken-for-granted aspects of the musicians' art, and they caused, at times, some difficulty for the musicians to express what was going on, not so much musically, but in terms of their embodied sense of the experience. Brian captures what many musicians would say when they were taking for granted their embodied sensations: "I don't know if I can explain that any more than I have." Though discussion stimulated them to describe it in more detail, the taken-for-grantedness of the event had them routinely accepting the magic moment as a part of their lifeworld without further explanation. The video review afforded them a rare opportunity to achieve clarity and consensus for their taken-for-granted, yet mysterious, embodied sensations.

A key requirement or convention in playing jazz music is the act of listening to understand the musical meaning of what is going on and responding in a meaningful way, which corresponds to the Schutzian idea of *wide-awakedness*, "a plane of consciousness of highest tension originating in an attitude of full attention to life and its requirements" (Schutz, 1973, 7, 213). Paul's (another study participant) description of playing with "ears wide open" captures this idea, as a typification of more than simply listening; it includes increased understanding and awareness of what is heard, and the act of responding appropriately, in a meaningful way.

Another taken-for-granted aspect of the musicians' lifeworld is the sense of time: "Standard time is the intersection between durée and cosmic time as the universal temporal structure of the intersubjective world" (Schutz, 1973, 230). The intersubjective, cosmic time of the setting up and participating in a musical performance at a certain hour, in a certain space, with a certain group of musicians and listeners, is contrasted with the intersubjective *durée* experienced by anyone in the music space who enters into the collaborative meaning-making of the magic moment.

The magic-moment experience is outside of the taken-for-granted lifeworld, as it happens so infrequently. It is an example of what Schutz describes as a "specific shock which compels us to break through the limits of this 'finite' province of meaning and to shift the accent to another one" (1973, 231). Musicians describe this shift as entering into a musical world of flowing ideas where the work is effortless and easy. They also describe the need to limit their acknowledgement of the event as it is happening, for fear of it slipping through their grasp. As magic-moment experiences accumulate, they begin to enter into that lifeworld pool of taken-for-granted experiences and become part of the musicians' natural attitude, what Paul described as sought-after, "that's what you live for" phenomena. Yet the magic moment is such a profound, *elusive* experience that the shock is never diminished when it occurs; "the bar just keeps getting raised."

Musicians use the term *elusive* because they see the magic moment as a state they cannot control or anticipate; if they try to "prime themselves" for it, it can "backfire." Two musicians in expressed it this way:

> *Sanchez*: It isn't something that you can predict. It doesn't always happen just because you want it to.

> *Joe*: I don't think that you can say "Okay, now let's try to create a zone of an altered state leading to an ecstatic moment."

THEMATIC PATTERNS TO MAGIC MOMENTS

In my research, musicians expressed the meaning of magic moments under the themes of the environment, cultural conventions, the self-other relationship, the body-mind, temporality-*durée*, the music itself, and technical competence-learning. For illustration here, I offer some of the more evocative findings embedded in the descriptions of the self-other relationship; the body-mind, specifically the de-afferentation process; and temporality.

Self-Other: Relationship Between Musicians

The most impactful factors in the creation of the magic-moment experience have to do with relationship between the self and other. Musicians have a strong need to establish and maintain a sense of trust in the group:

maintaining an appreciative atmosphere, supporting each other in the music even if disagreeing with musical decisions, building off of each others' ideas, and listening hard to what is going on in order to respond in meaningful ways and make musical sense of all of their simultaneous contributions. They use terms such as *in the pocket* and *in the zone* to signify a safe place where musicians are in sync. Several spoke of the trust necessary to be able to take risks and express themselves in the group. For Sanchez, trust means that "no one will be jumping on your back [if] something isn't exactly perfect. If the energy is kind and positive you can take down some of those walls." If trust is unavailable in the group, the expressive play cannot develop to a point of detachment, as the musicians are on guard or careful about what and how they play.

When trust is available, the in-the-moment, composed music is likened to a collaborative work of art, what Jack called a "sonic sculpture," that coalesces and is unified by the musician sculptors simultaneously adding their intimate expression, "feeding off of the other players a lot; picking up an idea and carrying something." For this to occur, each musician commits primarily to the group creation rather than his solo performance. There is a letting go of individual focus, and a mindful intentionality around collaboration.

> *Paul:* There is that integration with the other people. There is a responsiveness that is going on that makes it exciting. You are just careening all over the place and you don't know where you are going. You get jolts from the other musicians. You're suddenly stimulated.

The act of listening in performance is more than simply hearing a musical idea. The engaged listener is completely focused, validating the other's presence and value, embracing what the other is offering, and offering ideas that make sense. Musicians speak of different levels of listening and meaningful response:

> *Matt:* We were completely responding to one another's musical gestures, emotional gestures. There was a dissolving of boundaries, so the group became one unit in which everybody sort of melded together. There's a bonding that happens with the people involved. There's a recognition in a group that this is happening, which then circles back and amplifies the personal experience.

These musicians used the concept of *making sense* to discuss how they dealt with mistakes and navigated through tough spots. A couple of them disagreed with the concept of problem solving when describing what happens when they run into trouble: not working the situation as a problem, or describing what they do as *problem-making*, but describing it as a desire to continue making musical sense within the musical structure and within the collaborative sharing of musical ideas. It is a constant effort to move forward, responding to what is stated:

> *Paul*: You can't stop making sense. If you stop making sense, then your solo dies for that moment. Sometimes that can be a lot of fun, too, because it's the unexpected and you still have to be musical there.

The process of responding to others in an unself-conscious way, supporting and appreciating the expressive meaning-making, is what needs to happen for the whole group to, as Brian put it, "lock together," to entrain. Part of that entrainment has to do with similar competence levels on the instruments and proficiency in the music. But, that said, experienced musicians describe entrainment as more of a social process of opening up to the music and the musicians, listening really hard in order to connect, assertively responding, and contributing musical color, shape, and texture that makes sense with what is going on:

> *Matt*: [We] were very synched. I wasn't working at all to integrate that mix of sounds, and this tune clicked.

This is not to say that a less experienced musician couldn't contribute, but lack of experience often becomes a distraction to the others or requires the other musicians to pay more attention to managing the group sound. Further, if one or more members of the group is not listening, not committed to the collaboration, and contributes an idea that doesn't fit with the ideas that are currently expressed, the focus is interrupted, trust is violated, and the group members' awareness comes back into conscious focus:

> *Sanchez*: You could be playing something, and implying some sort of concept, and sense that another person is not really keyed into what you're doing. It's like getting interrupted in the middle of a sentence. It takes a while to get back to that place where you're not conscious of anything but the sound.

Even if the players are listening and engaged, they must delve deep to provide one another with meaningful and stimulating musical ideas. Each musician needs to contribute to the group composition, a compilation of individual musical personalities somehow melded together:

> *Matt*: Any exploratory moves that they make in terms of defining that harmonic shape is immediately responded to by the rest of the people, by going in a direction that is being suggested or responding some other way.

When each player assumes this responsibility and commitment, then no one player has to maintain conscious vigilance or assume the role of carrying anyone or propping them up, and all are free to let go and focus on their own contributions:

> Matt: People who are fully responsive, there's no differentiation. When the horn player begins to play, the way they are playing their eighth notes is integrated into the way the bass player is laying out the quarter notes and the way the drummer is riding on the cymbal. It's fundamental interactive dynamics that have to be here for me in order to get to that place.

There is an assortment of nonverbal, verbal, and musical cues used to convey energy and meaning between players, similar to conversation cues. Overt cues such as verbal direction, looks, nods, turns, embodied movement coordinated with the music, and emphasis within the musical structure are supplemented by more covert nuance conveyed through slight movement and embodied energy shifts. An example of this was noted in one videotaped session, wherein the alto saxophone player conveyed intensity through his solo (in tone, speed, and timbre) and his body (by rocking, lifting his head and sax, and moving his feet). The ensemble responded to the cues by playing with more intensity (a driving beat in the drums, an intense walking bass, and additional tones in the piano chording). This was also a point in the performance when the audience clearly refocused its attention on the group, applauded, and gave vocal reinforcement to the soloist.

The musicians described physical comfort emerging when playing with others who clicked, providing strong support. Dorell detailed how the group began to "feel its way" and find a "comfortable level" of rhythm and energy. Next, he described a "loosening up," at which point his hand motions became more fluid and he felt a "body shift" happening, which helped move him into more "interesting" play, more energy:

> Dorell: And, you could feel it build when it started to happen. And that was quite amazing. I can see it in my body, I can hear it in the sound, I can see it in the stretch.

Being One With the Music

There is an embodied sense that aligns the musician with the music, extending out through the instrument. Entrainment also occurs between musicians, uniting the collaboration into a seamless whole. The felt sense is an effortless flowing of and being one with the music at the same time. Musicians report feelings of detachment yet connectedness with other musicians and audience: ecstasy, bliss, music flowing through, thoughtless, relaxed, acute musical awareness, weightlessness, lightness of being, electricity, emotion, lack of emotion, even out-of-body experiences. For example, Brian spoke of his loss of the sense of a distinction between performer and audience. Each musician described the embodied sensations differently, but all agreed that the feelings start with detachment from the ego or self, musical awareness becomes more acute, and the embodied feelings are positive, intense, and different than the feelings or experiences in the day-to-day lifeworld.

> *Paul:* You are just on autopilot, and it's effortless, and your instrument is an extension of who you are. That's ecstasy. It's a spiritual experience. When everything is right . . . it's like out-of-body . . . you're just watching yourself, aware, musically what is happening around you. You are really aware of being part of it. You're not aware of any physical stress or physical tension or any physical interference or physical strain whatsoever. You're just sitting back, laying back, . . . seeing yourself play, . . . that complete detachment, . . . as if you are hovering.

Musicians describe facets of the music as critical to detachment. Contributing musical factors to this detachment include the beat and musical shapes, feeling like they become part of the body, causing involuntary movement and general entrainment.

> *Sanchez:* You just get into this rhythm, this dance, and you are very aware, very intimate with nature and a cycle.

> *Brian:* You're riding along on the line that the other person is playing, and the shape of the line will play out physically in your body.

The musicians unanimously agreed that, to experience the magic moment, they have to be in a relaxed state. There is minimal tension in the muscles and consciousness, and the problems and issues experienced in the day-to-day lifeworld are set outside of conscious awareness. This need for an embodied relaxation contrasts with the simultaneous need to be in an energetic state, keyed up with excitement and anticipation.

As the moment builds, the embodied energy also builds. One musician described the energy as coming through the music, the instrument, and his body. It builds up so much intensity that it feels as if the body moves without conscious control. He described it as a form of power, felt inside his body, that causes him to move. One of the drummers described a powerful light energy swirling in his torso, building as the music builds. Outward signs of this building energy include body movement such as rocking, lifting the knee, rising up from sitting, leaning forward or back, flushed face, expressive face, and changes in the musical color, shape, and texture.

Paul described a sense of disembodiment while in the magic moment, an "out-of-body" experience where he was sitting outside the group, watching himself and the other musicians' play, breaking free from the lifeworld, and experiencing what Husserl calls the *transcendental ego*.

> *Paul:* You're so detached, and it's so effortless, that it's almost as if you're watching it all unfold. You step back from the whole thing and take it in with extreme clarity. You don't always achieve that clarity because you're too involved, too attached.

Some of the musicians described feelings of levitating while experiencing a magic moment. They described a sense of lightness and weightlessness.

> *Brian:* You feel as if you are standing several inches off the ground. You could practically convince yourself, if you didn't look at your feet, that you're starting to pull up off of the floor.

A sax player thought it might be due to the wave of sound vibrations traveling through the body. A piano player described it as an overwhelming embodied energy coming from the music itself, the instrument, and energy coming from other musicians.

Temporality: *Durée*

Musicians are acutely aware of time, the outside, standard time, but more so, the inner time, or *durée*, intersected through bodily movement with standard time. Jazz music is unique because it is a simultaneous act of composing and performing. As Sanchez put it, "You play the notes and they're gone." The improvising musician cannot stop, back up, or rethink what is composed the way a painter or poet or scientist can. Jazz music is contained within the present and gone as musicians make musical choices while in *durée*. A common characteristic of the *magic-moment durée* is the sense that outside time slows or stands still, and inner time becomes the sense of the immediate moment and nothing else. Musicians indicated that it is very easy to experience a loss of outer time in a group situation or a solitary practice session:

> *Jack:* Your sphere of concentration becomes more Zen-like, where the past has very little to do with what you're doing. You have no thoughts of anything in the future.

The attractiveness of the *durée* for the musician has to do both with detaching from the outside world and immersing the self in the moment. A couple of the musicians described needing to extend solos long enough to get into a groove, to enter into the *durée*.

Each musician is responsible for keeping the time. This means that each is responsible for maintaining tempo (considered critical) and rhythm within the *durée*: maintaining a coordinated set of movements within the collaboration, and articulating the music within minimal tolerances:

> *Matt*: Playing jazz is always knowing where you are, where you've been, and where you're going. The only way that you could have all three of those perspectives is to have a detachment at the same time.

Thus, although they may not be cognizant of the past or the future within *durée*, the musicians hold the past and future as a non-conscious framework, active within the present.

TRANSFORMATIVE PHENOMENOLOGY: A PERSONAL REFLECTION

My underlying drive in this research was to explore the *magic-moment* phenomenon: to get at the underlying power and energy of this lived experience, to find out why it was and is such a compelling and addictive experience for me and these musicians. I now more clearly understand the meaning of the magic-moment experience, for not only my participant musicians but for myself. I understand the power of the magic-moment experience to provide a way to break free of the taken-for-granted lifeworld and cohabit an idyllic space with others.

The improvisation process can be applied in a variety of venues: in the arts, business, or any situation in which we engage in intense experience. Factors described as being instrumental to achieving a magic moment easily cross over into other domains. Relational factors of trust creation and acceptance of ideas promote a willingness to try new, less *safe* strategies. An initial focus on appreciative collaboration, rather than output, produces better outcomes.

An exciting and unanticipated outcome of this research has been its impact on my personal and professional life. Phenomenological method is similar to the act of improvisation, wherein my *self* strives for detachment yet, at the same time, my body-mind is coupling with the rhythms of the *other*. Phenomenology is much more than a method; it is a lifestyle, *a way of being in the world*. I find myself integrating these factors into my work and relationships, at times feeling totally engaged yet, at the same time, detached, observing the situation I am in. I am working to develop a mindfulness around deafferentation: opening myself up to the human rhythms and improvisations I find in my life and consulting practice. As I become more mindfully detached from my ego and preferred outcomes, I notice myself becoming more accepting and compassionate. This seems to influence others in their own acceptance and focus on collaborative outcomes.

It is difficult for me to determine which impacted me more—my research interests or the phenomenological method I used to analyze the data. I think both. To me, the acts of jazz improvisation and phenomenological practice have many process similarities. As I entered into the phenomenological research, I found comfort in the practice. It was as if I was coming home to a familiar neighborhood, with doors wide open, inviting me in, with plenty of jazz and open possibilities. While studying the academic language and phenomenological process, I began to realize that I had been practicing aspects of phenomenology since I was quite young, namely, focusing in the moment and setting my *self* outside of the situation, detached and observant, improvising, and searching for meaning. Studying the phenomenological method validated that lifestyle and transformed my practice.

My consulting practice has become richer as a result, another transformational realization. I fancy that I traverse my work using childlike eyes, aware of and bracketing my own filters and biases, while being completely *with* my client. Each bit of information discovered in dialogue must be considered new and relevant, perhaps another key to unlocking the underlying meaning that holds a client back from his own attempt to reach a magic moment. Data analysis, for me, is now much more complicated, yet natural and flowing, as I insert myself into the work with the client, cohabit the client story, work with "big ears," as a musician friend terms it; I live, I dance (van Manen, 2002), and I spiral with the client data (Bentz and Shapiro, 1998), to understand and find the underlying meaning of the phenomena. I invite my client to go down a phenomenological path with me, to sit with the data, and move from first- to second-order constructs (Schutz, 1953), uncovering relevant characteristics and building richer, more appreciative scenarios (Cooperrider, 1999).

Each client group and coaching session is another phenomenological opportunity to assertively make sense about what is going on in my work and in my life. I find that I do not need to be the expert, but more of a supportive partner inserting my *self* into the search together. Each slight act of risk-taking results in building more trust and sharing deeper, more vital and real data, and hence more impactful results. I work to get into a sort of rhythm with the client, coupling with them through empathy and vocal nuance.

Finally, I notice that I have more discomfort with our Western society's socially constructed norms about dialogue, where a common practice is to listen just long enough to draw conclusions based on limited data and assumptions, and then offer solutions, or argue, and move on. Time is rarely allowed, in business, to truly sit with information or dwell in the adaptive tension that would offer more opportunities for group engagement and determination of underlying meaning (Heifetz, 1994). On the other hand, my work with clients offers the chance to dwell phenomenologically with the data, to take the time to sit in a meaning-making space, and take the time to coax that meaning to the surface.

REFERENCES

Bentz, Valerie M., and Jeremy J. Shapiro. (1998) *Mindful Inquiry in Social Research.* Thousand Oaks, CA: Sage.

Bergson, Henri. (1913/2001). *Time and Free Will* (F. L. Pogson, Trans.). Mineola, NY: Dover.

———. (1998). *Creative Evolution* (A. Mitchell, Trans.). Mineola, NY: Dover.

Berliner, Paul F. (1994) *Thinking in Jazz: The Infinite Art of Improvisation.* Chicago: University of Chicago Press.

Cooperrider, David L. (1999) *Appreciative Inquiry: Rethinking Human Organization Toward a Positive Theory of Change.* Chicago: Stipes.

Cotterill, Rodney M. J. (1995) On the Unity of Conscious Experience. *Journal of Consciousness Studies, 2*(4), 290–312.

———. (1996) Prediction and Internal Feedback in Conscious Perception. *Journal of Consciousness Studies, 3*(3), 245–66.

———. (2001) Evolution, Cognition and Consciousness. *Journal of Consciousness Studies, 8*(2), 3–17.

Damasio, Antonio R. (1997) Towards a Neuropathology of Emotion and Mood. *Nature, 386*(6627), 769–71.

Depraz, Natalie. (1999) The Phenomenological Reduction as Praxis. In F. J. Varela and J. Shear (Eds.), *The View from Within: First Person Approaches to the Study of Consciousness* (95–110). London: Imprint Academic.

Gallese, Vittorio. (2001) The "Shared Manifold" Hypothesis. *Journal of Consciousness Studies, 8*(5–7), 33–50.

Gass, Susan M., and Alison Mackey. (2000) *Stimulated Recall Methodology in Second Language Research.* Mahwah, NJ: Lawrence Erlbaum.

Greeley, Andrew M. (1974) *Ecstasy: A Way of Knowing.* Englewood Cliffs, NJ: Prentice-Hall.

Grime, Kitty. (1983) *Jazz Voices.* New York: Quartet Books.

Heifetz, Ronald A. (1994) *Leadership Without Easy Answers.* Cambridge, MA: Belknap Press of Harvard University Press.

Jeddeloh, Steven. (2001) The Future of Leadership: Continuous Transformation. In W. Hammond, III (Ed.), *12 Step Wisdom at Work: Transforming Your Life and Your Organization* (300). London: Kogan Page.

———. (2003) Chasing Transcendence: Experiencing "Magic Moments" in Jazz Improvisation. Unpublished Ph.D. Dissertation. Santa Barbara, CA: Fielding Graduate Institute.

Laski, Marghanita. (1961) *Ecstasy in Secular and Religious Experiences.* Los Angeles: Jeremy P. Tarcher.

Leonard, Neil (1987) *Jazz: Myth and Religion*. New York: Oxford University Press.

Monson, Ingrid (1996) *Saying Something: Jazz Improvisation and Interaction*. Chicago: University of Chicago Press.

Newberg, Andrew, and Eugene G. D'Aquili. (2000) The Neuropsychology of Religious and Spiritual Experience. In J. Anderson and R. K. C. Forman (Eds.), *Cognitive Maps and Spiritual Maps* (251–66). Charlottesville, VA: Imprint Academic.

Rehorick, David A. (1986) Shaking the Foundations of the Lifeworld: A Phenomenological Account of an Earthquake Experience. *Human Studies, 9*, 379–91.

Roy, Louis. (2001) *Transcendent Experiences: Phenomenology and Critique*. Toronto, Ontario, Canada: University of Toronto Press.

Schon, Donald. (1983) *The Reflective Practitioner*. New York: Basic Books.

Schutz, Alfred. (1953) Common-Sense and Scientific Interpretation of Human Action. *Philosophy and Phenomenological Research, XIV*(1), 1–38.

———. (1967) *The Phenomenology of the Social World* (F. G. a. L. Walsh, Trans.). Evanston, IL: Northwestern University Press.

———. (1973). *Collected Papers I: The Problem of Social Reality*. The Hague, The Netherlands: Martinus Nijhoff.

Schutz, Alfred, and Thomas Luckmann. (1973) *The Structures of the Life-World* (R. M. Zaner and H. T. Engelhardt, Trans.). Evanston, IL: Northwestern University Press.

van Manen, Max (Ed.). (2002) *Writing in the Dark: Phenomenological Studies in Interpretive Inquiry*. London, Ontario, Canada: Althouse Press.

Wallace, B. Alan. (1999) The Buddhist Tradition of Samatha: Methods for Refining and Examining Consciousness. In F. J. Varela and J. Shear (Eds.), *The View from Within: First Person Approaches to the Study of Consciousness* (175–87). London: Imprint Academic.

Zaner, Richard M. (1981) *The Context of Self: A Phenomenological Inquiry Using Medicine as a Clue*. Athens: Ohio University Press.

Index

artists, case study of applied
phenomenology, 195–203
autobiographical accounts, 55
autoethnography and phenomenology,
98–99

Backhaus, Gary, xx
Behnke, Elizabeth, 22, 142
Bentz, Valerie Malhotra, 3–4, 7, 8–9,
12–13, 15, 17–18, 20, 22, 23–24,
26n1, 27n5, 51, 52, 53, 55, 56, 70,
84, 104, 115, 117, 131, 143, 172,
221. *See also* Malhotra, Valerie
body: and disability, 181; and Eastern
practices, 143, 187; and feminism,
181; phenomenology of, 7,
217–19; in scholarship, 84;
source of knowledge, 34–37,
84, 101, 107, 141–42, 172;
tracking symptoms, 33; as
traitorous, 84. *See also* embodied;
embodiment
bodymindfulness, 142–43; cultivation
of, 149–50, 151; as energetic
presence, 143
bodymindset, 142, 145; shifting,
147–48; themes, 152

bracketing, 11–14, 20; cross-cultural,
143; defined, 189n1; disabilities as
natural brackets, 13; examples of,
197; McGrane experiment, 177, 184,
187; transcendental, 13–14
breast cancer, 83–84; fear of, 85–89;
limitation of clinical studies, 90. *See
also* cancer; cancer survivor
breathing: deep, 149, 175; in tai chi,
182–83

cancer: depression as cancer patient,
67, 76–77; as long-term journey, 72,
80; and phenomenology, 70; social
context, 89; treatment, 74–76. *See
also* breast cancer; cancer survivor
cancer survivor, 67–69;
transformational experience of, 69;
transformation themes and stages,
72–79. *See also* breast cancer; cancer
coaching: phenomenology and, 205,
220–21; and protocols, 206
conscientización, 157, 171;
consciousness development in
Latinas, 168–72
consciousness: development in Latinas,
168–72; embodied, 183, 209;

prereflective, 184; theory development, 169–72; and wide-awakedness, 213. *See also* intentionality

consulting practice, informed by phenomenology, 221–22. *See also* coaching

couvade: defined, 37–40; empirical studies, 40–41; necessity of phenomenological approach, 45–46; reconceptualization, 42–44; ritual, 37; symptoms of, 38–41; syndrome, 37–47

descriptions: and bracketing, 12; commonsense typifications, 212; of embodied empathic resonance, 150–51; as essential to phenomenology, 6, 10–12, 35–36, 46, 115, 122–24, 177, 208; hermeneutics of Gadamer, 20–21; Husserlian and Schutzian, 25; increased awareness, 144, 148; of Latinas' experience, 157, 161; opposed to biomedical language, 85; overlapping in meaning, 212; as protocols, 131, 195. *See also* phenomenological research

disabilities as natural brackets, 13

disruption of mundane reality, 184–86

dissonance and consonance: essence of, 167–69; experience of, 147, 151–53

dogmatism, phenomenology as antidote to, 19–20

dualism, phenomenology as antidote to, 7, 91

durée and time in jazz, 209, 213–14, 219–20

earthquakes: experience of, 15; phenomenological interpretation of, 5, 177–78; questions elicited by wonderment of, 6; typifications of, 18

eidetic phenomenology, 8, 11, 25; eidetic reduction characterized, 210;

eidetic reduction and mindfulness, 210

embodied: consciousness aspect, 25; empathic resonance, 143–46, 150–53; experience of jazz musicians, 212–19; the "I" as embodied, 179–89, 189n1; Latinas' consciousness, 168; wisdom, 172; wonderment, 34–36; writing, 13

embodiment, 9, 46, 89–91, 151; defined, 83–86; as gendered, 188; in tai chi, 180–83

Embree, Lester, 6

emotions: alienation, 73; anger, 130, 168, 171; anxiety in researcher, 47, 58–60; consonance and dissonance, 151–52; in couvade, 34–35, 37–40; depression as cancer patient, 67, 76–77; ecstasy, 208; existential terror, 68, 73–74, 207; of expectant fathers, 43, 46; fear, 59, 71, 83–89, 100–101, 124–25; grief and pain, 169; love, 76, 78, 208; pleasure of discovery in phenomenology, 54; pleasure and success, 147; push-pull in learning phenomenology, 21, 23, 54; release, 208

empirical studies: assumptions underlying, 44–45; and couvade research, 40–41; and phenomenology, 34, 45–46

energetic presence, 148–49, 151

epoche of everyday life, suspension, 187, 209–10

ethnic identity, 165–67

ethnomethodology, development from phenomenology, 7

experience, tracking, 33

Fielding Graduate University, 4, 67, 194. *See also* scholar-practitioners

fundamental anxiety. *See* Schutz, Alfred

Gadamer, Hans-Georg, 8, 20–21, 27nn3–4, 131–38

Garfinkel, Harold, 7, 177

Giorgi, Amedeo, 6

reality: mundane, disruption of, 184–86; paramount, of everyday life, 4, 181

reflection: as key to transformation, 75; mental and embodied, 181

Rehorick, David, 4, 5, 9–11, 14, 15, 17, 18, 22, 26n1, 33–36, 46, 51, 84, 177, 178, 181, 183

relationships: after cancer, 67–68; business, trouble in, 194; in couvade, 40–46; to death, 101; in jazz, 210, 214–17; kidney donor-recipient, 95; Latinas, 167; renewed through phenomenology, 206; revitalization of, 185–86; as text, 8; we-relationships among jazz musicians, 189

relevance: significance of, 18–20; and typifications, 17–20. *See also* typifications

research participants, transformation of, 72, 78, 139, 172, 201–3, 205–6

Ricoeur, Paul, 10, 27n3, 70

scholar-practitioners, 4–5, 23–24, 26, 45

Schutz, Alfred, 4, 8, 10, 17–20, 25, 55, 115, 117–18, 122, 126–27, 178–82, 183, 184, 185, 186, 187, 189, 190n2, 209, 211–12, 213–14, 221; first- and second-order constructs, 177, 221; on fundamental anxiety, 19, 178–79; and Luckmann, 179–80, 213; stocks of knowledge, 185; typifications, 8–9; we-relationship, 209, 211–12. *See also* lifeworld

Schwartz, Michael, 19

Shapiro, Jeremy, 3–4, 9, 15, 17–18, 20, 23–24, 27n5, 51, 52, 53, 56, 70, 84, 104, 115, 117, 131, 143, 221

social phenomenology applied, 10–11

social sensitivity, 182, 185, 190n2. *See also* habituation

somatic epistemology, 152

spirituality, 60–61, 79, 160–61, 208

stress, 218; and cancer, 71–78; in couvade, 38

symptoms: attunement, 42; as compathetic response, 43; sympathetic response to pregnancy, 35–36; sympathetic and unrecognized, 33, 36–37

tai chi: cognitive reflection, 182; learning, 176, 182–83, 186–87; and phenomenology, 187–89; and temporality, 183

techniques in phenomenology, 144. *See also* bracketing; horizontalization; imaginative variations

thematic analysis, examples of, 34–35, 58–62, 72–79, 159–67, 199, 214–20

theory in the flesh, of Latinas, 157, 169, 172

time and *durée* in jazz, 209, 213–14, 219–20

transcendence, 179; characterized, 208; and flow, 186; and immanence, 179; transcendencies, 179–81, 183

transcendental ego, in jazz and Husserl, 219

transformation. *See* phenomenological researcher; research participants

transformative phenomenologists, 4–5. *See also* phenomenological researcher

transformative phenomenology, 5; applications, 25–26; cultivating phronesis, 24–25; four founders, 6–8; Husserl on, 26; as jazz improvisation, 220–22; as wild horse, 21, 25

typifications, 8, 13; defined and applied, 17–20, 180, 184; of earthquake, 18; evoking, 35, 188; to maintain normalcy, 213; and musical performance, 212; and relevance, 18–20; Schutz, 8–9

About the
Editors and Contributors

Valerie Malhotra Bentz, Ph.D., (Editor) is professor of human and organization development at Fielding Graduate University, where she also served as associate dean for research. She taught in the doctoral program in sociology at Texas Woman's University for twelve years. Her books include *Mindful Inquiry in Social Research* (with Jeremy Shapiro, 1998) and *Becoming Mature: Childhood Ghosts and Spirits in Adult Life* (1989). She is a fellow in contemplative practice of the American Association of Learned Societies, and consulting research professor in somatic psychology at the Santa Barbara Graduate Institute. Dr. Bentz was editor of *Phenomenology and the Human Sciences* (1994–1998). She has served as president and board member of the Clinical Sociology Association and the Sociological Practice Association. She founded and co-directed an action research team and center in Mizoram, India. Valerie was co-founder of the Creative Longevity and Wisdom Initiative at Fielding. She has experience as a practitioner of psychotherapy, yoga instruction, certified massage therapy, and body-spirit integration. Her current interests include sociological theory, consciousness development, Vedantic and Buddhist theories of knowledge, and social somatics. She has written a philosophical novel, and plays piano and bassoon.

Gloria L. Córdova, Ph.D., is an independent consultant, facilitator, personal coach, and speaker. Her work in phenomenology and critical Chicana feminist theory raises consciousness in the reclamation and reconstruction of personal and ethnic identity. Dr. Córdova uses narratives, storytelling, and writing as tools to analyze and interpret these phenomena. She is an award-winning professional speaker and advocate for women and minorities. An avid genealogy researcher, Dr. Córdova pursues family history research with a commitment to finding and honoring her Spanish-Mexican heritage.

Lucy Dinwiddie, Ph.D., is vice-president of organization development at ConAgra Foods, in Omaha, Nebraska. She held prior positions as director of organization development at Ford Motor Company and EDS, and senior manager at Ernst and Young. Dr. Dinwiddie is a certified clinical sociologist and executive coach. She earned a master of science in organizational development from American University, and a master of arts in human development and doctorate in human and organizational systems from Fielding Graduate University.

David B. Haddad, Ph.D., is an executive coach, management consultant, and social researcher. Prior to obtaining his doctorate from Fielding Graduate University, he was a financial and investment professional with Fidelity Investments. He brought balance to his Wall Street background with nonprofit leadership in neighborhood housing revitalization, having served as finance director of an agency serving two Michigan counties. Now living in Carlsbad, California, Dr. Haddad is a teacher of spirituality, healing, apologetics, and church history. His research interests include Husserlian phenomenology, action research, and the structure of social research methodologies.

Steven C. Jeddeloh, Ph.D., is a leadership consultant with over twenty years' experience helping individuals and organizations strive for optimal performance. He serves as adjunct faculty at Capella University. Dr. Jeddeloh has been a musician, business leader, small business owner, human resources manager, and consultant. He has co-authored a variety of published training manuals, and is the author of "The Future of Leadership," a chapter in *The Twelve Steps of Leadership*. Dr. Jeddeloh earned master's degrees from the University of Minnesota in both education and organizational development, and a doctorate in human and organizational systems from Fielding Graduate University.

Marc J. LaFountain, Ph.D., is professor of sociology at the University of West Georgia, where he teaches courses on phenomenological sociology, visual sociology, sociology of emotions and the body, and critical theory. He also serves as program coordinator for the interdisciplinary environmental studies program. His book, *This is Not an Essence: Dali and Postmodernism*, was published by SUNY Press (1997). His research and publications have appeared in a wide array of disciplines, including sociology, psychology, philosophy, communications, and art and literary criticism. Dr. LaFountain's work has appeared in *Human Studies, Critical Studies in Mass Communication, Humanity & Society,* and *The Humanistic Psychologist.* Currently, he is exploring issues on the body and cultural politics.

Adair Linn Nagata, Ph.D., is professor of intercultural communication at the Rikkyo University Graduate School of Intercultural Communication in Tokyo. She also teaches at the Graduate School of Asia-Pacific Studies at Waseda University. Her career has spanned international education and corporate training, communication, and organizational development in a global financial services company. She earned a master's degree in education from Harvard University, and a doctorate in human development from Fielding Graduate University. Her publications focus on the cultivation of consciousness and communicative competence in intercultural relationships. Her scholarly and teaching activities emphasize a pedagogy that encourages integrative transformative learning in intercultural education, and applications of conceptions such as bodymindfulness and mindful inquiry.

Jeffrey Nonemaker, Ph.D., who earned his doctorate in human and organizational systems from Fielding Graduate University, is director of international student recruitment and admissions at the University of La Verne in California. His research has focused on applied social phenomenology related to organ donation. He was a review editor of the *Journal of the Association of American International Colleges and Universities.* Jeffrey served as the chief academic officer for the University of La Verne's Athens, Greece, campus from 1983 until 2004.

Bernie Novokowsky, Ph.D., is a senior organizational effectiveness and management consultant based in Calgary, Alberta, Canada. Dr. Novokowsky completed his Ph.D. in human and organizational systems at Fielding Graduate University in 1998. Over the past fourteen years, he has been consultant to executives and managers in over 120 companies, spanning the international corporate, public, and not-for-profit sectors. Dr. Novokowsky has offered workshops and seminars at the University of Calgary and the Banff School of Management. As a scholar-practitioner, he seeks to apply insights from hermeneutic phenomenology to transform individual, group, and organizational life.

Linda Susan Trewin Nugent, Ph.D., is professor of nursing at the Saint John campus of the University of New Brunswick in Canada. Through the unique lens of a nurse-sociologist, her research on home care has developed from her experiences as a family member and professional nurse. Dr. Nugent has explored the support needs of family caregivers, and examined the structure and processes involved in the labor of home support workers.

She has received support and funding from the Medical Research Fund of the New Brunswick provincial government. Her current focus of inquiry is an exploration of the support service needs of senior citizens who reside in rural communities.

David Allan Rehorick, Ph.D., (Senior Editor) is professor emeritus of sociology at the University of New Brunswick (UNB), Canada, where he taught from 1974 to 2007. Currently, he is professor of human and organization development at Fielding Graduate University. His research, publications, and editorial contributions encompass the domains of applied social phenomenology, cross-cultural educational praxis, sociological theory, the healthcare sciences, and the creative arts. He has served on six journal editorial boards, including review editor of *Human Studies: A Journal for Philosophy and the Social Sciences.* Dr. Rehorick was appointed founding faculty and fellow of comparative culture at the Miyazaki International College in Japan (1994–1998). He was a developer, teacher, and first director of international internships at Renaissance College, the first undergraduate studies program in Canada (2000–2004). Dr. Rehorick is an award-winning educator and teacher. At UNB, he was appointed university teaching scholar (2005–2008), and received the Allan P. Stuart Memorial Award for Excellence in Teaching (1984). He received national recognition with the Association of Atlantic Universities Instructional Leadership Award (1995). He plays jazz piano, and is studying the intersection of language, consciousness, and music.

Sandy Simpson, Ph.D., earned her doctorate at Fielding Graduate University, and is currently a psychology instructor at the University of Central Florida. She works with undergraduates and clinical psychology master's degree students. Her professional experience includes a private psychotherapy practice and psychological work in a forensic setting. She applies her interest in phenomenology by introducing phenomenological philosophy and encouraging her students to interpret the experiences of their own lives and learning. Dr. Simpson and her husband, Bob Pritchard, live in Orlando, Florida. They enjoy sea and river kayaking, wilderness hiking, and playing in the ocean with their two grandchildren.

Roanne Thomas-MacLean, Ph.D., is assistant professor in the department of sociology at the University of Saskatchewan, Canada. Prior to this appointment, she completed a postdoctoral fellowship in interdisciplinary primary healthcare research. Her interests focus on the exploration of chronic illness, particularly cancer, and its implications for people's everyday lives. She holds a Canadian Institutes of Health Research/Saskatchewan

Health Research Foundation New Investigator Award in support of her research activities.

Dudley O. Tower, Ph.D., is a fellow in creative longevity and wisdom at Fielding Graduate University, where he earned his doctorate in 2000. Dr. Tower has extensive experience as an organizational consultant and a psychotherapist. His experience with life-threatening cancer in 1988 led to a reassessment and transformation of his life, one that entailed ending a career as chief financial officer for a major automotive company. He is currently living happily in Landrum, South Carolina, where he teaches and contributes to the administration of a lifelong learning program at Furman University in Greenville.

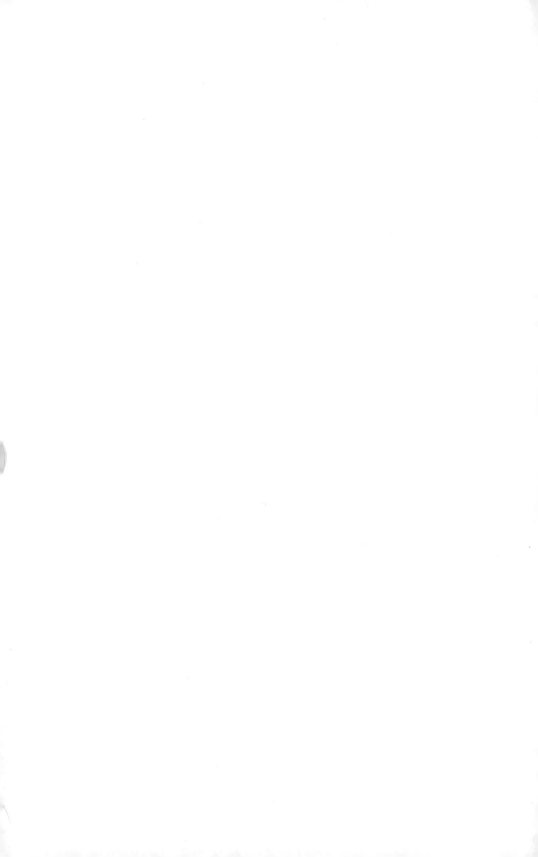

Made in the USA
Lexington, KY
17 July 2012